Intermittent Fasting and Ketogenic Diet:

Lose weight, feel energetic and be healthy with keto-intermittent fasting +7 Day Keto Meal Plan for women and men to maximize fat loss

Tim Martin

The follow Book is reproduced below with the goal of providing information that is as accurate and reliable as possible. Regardless, purchasing this Book can be seen as consent to the fact that both the publisher and the author of this book are in no way experts on the topics discussed within and that any recommendations or suggestions that are made herein are for entertainment purposes only. Professionals should be consulted as needed prior to undertaking any of the actions endorsed herein.

This declaration is deemed fair and valid by both the American Bar Association and the Committee of Publishers Association and is legally binding throughout the United States.

Furthermore, the transmission, duplication or reproduction of any of the following work including specific information will be considered an illegal act irrespective of whether it is done electronically or in print. This extends to creating a secondary or tertiary

Table of Contents

Introduction

Intermittent fasting and the ketogenic diet are akin to those peanut butter cups that you will be put aside once and for all once you get started, they are two great tastes that taste even better together.

The following chapters will discuss everything you need to know not just about the ketogenic diet and intermittent fasting, but why they work so well together and how to maximize the effectiveness of each in order to turn your body into a lean, mean, fat-burning machine while helping you to look and feel better than you have in years in the process.

There are plenty of books on this subject on the market, thanks again for choosing this one! Every effort was made to ensure it is full of as much useful information as possible, please enjoy!

Chapter 1:

The Keto Diet Explained

Before carbohydrates were distressingly readily available, early humans had to rely on something else to create the energy they needed. As such, the liver is designed to produce a type of energy known as ketones when the right conditions are met. While most people don't typically take advantage of this ability, instead preferring to get their energy from the glucose found in carbohydrates, you can still access your liver's ability to produce energy while at the same time losing weight and feeling better than you likely have in years.

Weight loss naturally kicks into overdrive when the body enters a state of ketosis (it's ketone producing state) as the first thing the liver does is to break down any excess fat that it may currently be holding on to. Ketosis naturally occurs if you go without consuming enough daily calories for a prolonged period of time, but it can also be triggered by dropping your daily net carbohydrate intake to under 15 grams per day. Your net carbohydrate intake is simply the number of carbohydrates you consume in a day minus the amount of fiber you consume in the same 24-hour period.

Many diets today are just fads, but the ketogenic diet has been around for a long time. It may seem like something new that you have come across on the internet, but it was actually developed in the 1920's. At the Mayo Clinic in Minnesota, a doctor named R.M. Wilder was looking for ways to treat patients who suffered from seizures. In his research, he discovered the ketogenic way of eating and used it to treat his patients.

During the same era, the ketogenic diet was being pioneered by researchers in pediatric epilepsy at Johns Hopkins in Baltimore. The ketogenic diet proved successful at working miracles for these patients, and it was beloved for a period of time. Eventually, however, anti-seizure medications were introduced to treat patients; and for most people, taking a pill is far easier than completely changing the way you eat. The ketogenic diet was all but forgotten for decades.

Then, in 1994, Jim Abraham (the Hollywood film director) did an interview about his son Charlie on *Dateline NBC*. Abraham's son Charlie suffered from severe seizures. They had tried many forms of treatment, including all the seizure medications to no avail. When nothing else worked, Abraham sought different answers.

In his search to help his son, Abraham rediscovered the ketogenic diet that had been pioneered decades before. The Abraham family started following a ketogenic diet, and soon Charlie was living life seizure-free. Since the ketogenic diet reappeared on the healthy eating scene in the 1990s it has become increasingly popular both for those who are looking for an alternative to traditional seizure treatment as well as an excellent way to lose weight.

Ketogenic diet versus more traditional diets: To understand what makes the keto diet so very effective, it helps to take a look at a more traditional diet first as the differences will be readily visible. Most diets promote weight loss in a way that is the opposite of how the keto diet works and being prepared for these differences is sure to make your time with the keto diet even more effective.

While the keto diet focuses extensively on the types of foods that you eat, a more traditional diet focuses on limiting calories without spending too much time worrying about just what it is that is accounting for that number. Reducing the number of calories that you eat in a day will certainly decrease weight gain, but it is really only a temporary solution to a much larger issue.

As the average diet contains lots of carbs, some protein, and a little healthy fat, this leaves the body with no choice but to burn carbohydrates for fuel. This results in glucose being released into the system which is then broken down into a molecule known as ATP, which is the molecule that powers most traditional cell functions.

As ATP is created, insulin is also generated as a byproduct which goes on to affect your body in many different ways, some good and some bad. First, it helps ATP move throughout the body and also helps with storing the leftovers. Due to the fact that the average western diet is loaded with carbs, however, this excess is never brought out of cold storage which means it eventually just turns to fat instead. Again, as the average diet doesn't do anything to actively disrupt this cycle, it will, at best, curb excessive weight gain without doing anything to really get to the root of the issue.

It is also worth noting that the body's ability to burn fat effectively is limited while insulin is moving through your system. As such, it takes about eight hours from the last time you consumed carbs in excess for the body to return to a base state where it is ready to burn fat as effectively as possible once more. Rather than trying to lose weight when the deck is stacked against you, adopting the keto diet allows you to work with your body's natural process with the end result being that you will look and feel better than you ever imagined was possible.

Unlike these diets, the keto diet cuts right to what is really causing the issue and limits you to no more than 15 net grams of carbs per day. Once you reach a state of ketosis, your body will also begin a secondary process called lipolysis which is used to break down the fat in the body into a pair of molecules, fatty acid, and glycerol. The fatty acid is then used directly in the production of ketones as the liver takes it in and produces ketones in response. Ketones are then used for a vast majority of the processes that glucose typically powers; when they aren't enough, such as when the brain needs energy, glycerol is used instead.

Before making any serious changes to your regular diet, it is recommended that you always check with a dietitian or registered health care professional first to ensure that you won't end up causing yourself more harm than good on accident. If you are considering the ketogenic diet, then roughly 70 percent of what you eat moving forward should be comprised of healthy fat, with 25 percent dedicated to protein and 5 percent left over for carbohydrates. Those carbohydrates should primarily come from dairy, vegetables or nuts, no starch or wheat allowed. Each meal should be comprised of lots of natural healthy fats, a lean protein and lots of leafy, dark green vegetables.

Keto benefits

Once you have reached the required level of carbs and maintained for at least a week, your body will burn through its stores of glucose and start activating core ketogenic processes. The liver then breaks down stored fat into a pair of molecules, fatty acid, and glycerol. Fatty acids are what makes it possible for the body to create ketones in the first place, while the glycerol fills in for the glucose in specific instances where the ketones can't provide what the body needs. One such part of the body is the brain as it creates energy through what is known as gluconeogenesis.

While working to literally melt the fat off your body is a great start, there are numerous additional benefits when it comes to remaining in the ketogenic state for a prolonged period of time. What's more, the longer the state persists, the more pronounced the positive effects become.

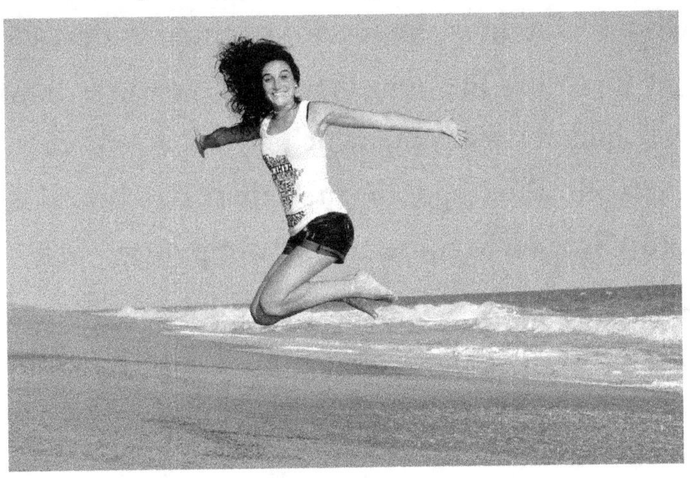

Improves immune system: Aside from what it is capable of doing to your overall level of hunger, the ketogenic state is known to dramatically reduce the likelihood of numerous major health issues, starting with all of the types of cancer that are known to feed on glucose directly. While healthy cells can easily switch to burning ketones for energy, cancer cells are not that lucky which means they grow significantly more slowly than they otherwise would when deprived of their primary food source.

Switching to the keto diet is also ideal when it comes to promoting brain health for several reasons. The most important of these is the fact that following the keto diet is closer to the way early humans likely ate which means it is more in line with the type of fuel that the brain is naturally used to consuming. This, in turn, makes it possible for the brain to continue working at maximum capacity for longer than would otherwise be the case.

While it's true that the brain requires glucose to work properly, this is definitely the case of potentially having too much of a good thing. In this instance, if the brain receives too much glucose on a regular basis, then over time it will develop a higher tolerance which means that it will need to work harder in order to generate the same results. If left untreated this can lead to a state of glucose deprivation which can eventually lead to dementia. Utilizing glycerol as a replacement for glucose can then make it easier for the brain to function in the long-term without having to worry about these types of adverse effects, meaning that it is far more likely that degradation will occur.

Decreases hunger: Beyond simply helping you to burn fat more effectively, following a keto diet is also a great way to lose weight for a number of other reasons, starting with the fact that remaining in ketosis is actually proven to help you to remain feeling full after a meal far longer than would otherwise be the case. This is simply due to the fact that fat is more difficult to process than carbs which means your body won't begin to send out signals saying it is hungry until everything has been completely processed.

Additionally, while you can expect some carb cravings during the early part of ketosis, you will find that after you make it past this hurdle you will be able to remove food from your thoughts more easily than before. This is thanks to a useful hormone known as cholecystokinin which is the natural counter to ghrelin, the hormone responsible for telling you when you are hungry. Cholecystokinin is created by the body when food is moving through the intestines, but if you are in ketosis then it will be created at all times instead. The increased cholecystokinin production will continue for the full time your body remains in a ketogenic state, and even for a few days after you have left it.

What's more, besides making you look and feel better, the keto diet will also help you to feel fuller, longer and after eating a smaller serving of food. This is a natural side effect of a high fat and protein diet as both of these will stick with you much longer than any type of carbohydrates will. What's more, after you have entered a ketogenic state then your body will naturally start by burning visceral fat which is primarily fat that is stored in the midsection. All in all, a ketogenic state creates a scenario where your chance of heart disease decreases while your level of positive cholesterol increases. It is also known to reduce your risk of stroke and various other cardiovascular issues.

Chapter 2:

Getting Started

Once you have decided to truly embrace the potential of the keto diet, the first thing that you are going to need to be aware of is that the early days are going to be extremely tough going. This is completely natural, however, as your body has had years and years and years to develop new ways to break down carbs to produce energy but has no way to deal with burning fat ready to go on standby. As such, you are going to need to power through the time where your body doesn't have the fuel it is used to and is just working out how to access the fuel that is available to it. If you do manage to make it through, however, the natural benefits of ketosis will kick in and you are sure to feel that it was all worth it.

Starting ketosis: While it would be nice if it were not the case, there is more to getting started in ketosis than skipping carbs for a few meals. Rather, it is likely to take about a week for your body to start producing the ketones you need on a wide enough scale that you start to feel like your old self again. During this time, you are likely to experience a host of flu-like symptoms in addition to a severe lack of energy and general lack of motivation.

Cramps are common when beginning a keto diet. It's only minor but is very painful. It is due to mineral loss, especially magnesium because of greater urination. These are some ways to avoid it:

! Consume lots of salt and water. This will cut down on your magnesium loss and will help you avoid leg cramps.

! Supplement with magnesium, if you need to. Take three slow release magnesium tablets every day for 20 days. Then switch to one pill a day.

! If these steps don't help, you might have to increase your intake of carbs slightly. This will likely get rid of the issue. Watch your carbs, so you won't impact the diet.

Constipation is another side effect when first trying the keto diet since the digestive system will have to adapt. These are some ways to make the issue more manageable:

! Drink lots of water and consume salt. The most common reason for constipation is dehydration. Your body will remove the water from your colon causing the contents to become drier and harder, causing constipation. The solution would be drinking water and adding salt.

! Eat vegetables or other sources of fiber. Making sure you consume enough fiber from your diet will keep you regular. This will reduce your risk of constipation. This is a challenge with the low carb diet as many fiber sources are forbidden. Eating lots of non-starchy vegetables can help to add more fiber. Psyllium seed husks are water soluble and are a carb-free option.

! If all these steps don't help you can consume Milk of Magnesia to help with constipation.

Bad breath will let you know your body is burning fat and converting fat into ketones, which are fueling the brain. This smell may be noticed in body odor as well, especially if you sweat or work out a lot. Not everyone who eats a keto diet will experience bad breath. It is temporary and will go away in a few weeks. Once the body adapts, it will stop leaking the ketones through your sweat and breath.

While the going is going to be rough, you are going to want to keep in mind that what you are doing is exceedingly necessary and that if you give in to the temptation to indulge in your desire for carbs you will only be harming yourself as you will be prolonging the state before your body can properly enter ketosis.

During this period, you may find that adding a small fourth meal between lunch and dinner helps to negate the worst of the effects. If that doesn't help, consider the fact that every time your stomach growls you are actively moving towards ketosis and keep this in mind when the going gets exceptionally rough. During this period, you are going to want to limit yourself to 15 grams of carbohydrates per day, maximum, if you hope to reach your goal.

Track yourself: While waiting to hit the magic point of ketosis, it is important to test yourself during the transition phase to ensure you are on the right track. What you are going to test yourself for is a substance known as acetone which is a byproduct of breaking a ketone down into energy. While you can purchase blood tests or urine testing strips, there are also easier ways to test for ketosis. Specifically, you will know that you have reached a point of ketosis once your breath begins to smell like apples that are a few days too ripe and begins to taste more metallic on your tongue.

When it comes to ensuring your time spent on the ketogenic diet is as fruitful as possible it is important to work to fine-tune your ketosis level which means you will need to purchase what is known as a blood meter to check your ketone levels or you can use urine strips or a breath analyzer. Ideally, you will want a ketone level to beat anywhere from 3 and .5 millimolar to maximize your weight loss goals.

If, after testing yourself you find that your ketone level is still less than .5 millimolar then your body is not yet in a state of full ketosis which means you might want to cut your carbohydrates slightly more than what is outlined below. If you are somewhere between 1.5 ketones and .5 ketones, then your body is in the early stages of ketosis which is right where you want to be during weeks 1 and 2. If your ketone number ever rises above 3, however, then this is a sign that you are not consuming enough calories in a day.

The simplest, easiest and cheapest way to measure ketosis is with urine strips. For most beginners, this is a great first option. All you need to do is pee on the stick or dip it in your urine, and the color changes 15 seconds later. The color change will tell you if there is a presence of ketones or not. A dark purple reading shows that you are in ketosis.

Ketone Urine strips are great because they are available in any regular pharmacies and they are very cheap. However, the bad side of using urine strips is largely dependent on the amount of water you drink before you do the test.

Because of this, the pieces do not show a precise level of ketones. Also, as you go on with this diet, you will be more keto-adapted, and your body will then reabsorb the ketones from the using preventing the urine strips from effectively detecting the ketones even when you are already in ketosis.

Another simple way to measure ketones is using the breath analyzer. They are more expensive than the urine strips, starting at about $150. However, they are much cheaper than the meters. These analyzers are reusable many more times and work using a color code as well, as opposed to giving you a numerical value on the precise ketone level. The not very good thing about the breath analyzer is that it does not always correlate with blood ketone levels. It can sometimes show entirely misleading values.

Acceptable foods

Protein: As you are only going to want to ensure that only 25 percent of your caloric intake comes from protein, it is best to choose the right types. First, it is important to keep in mind that many proteins aren't actually good for you, especially those that are not certified as organic. Non-organic protein is prone to contain steroids as well as bacteria, neither of which your body needs. This is what makes grass-fed, locally grown and certified organic meat so important.

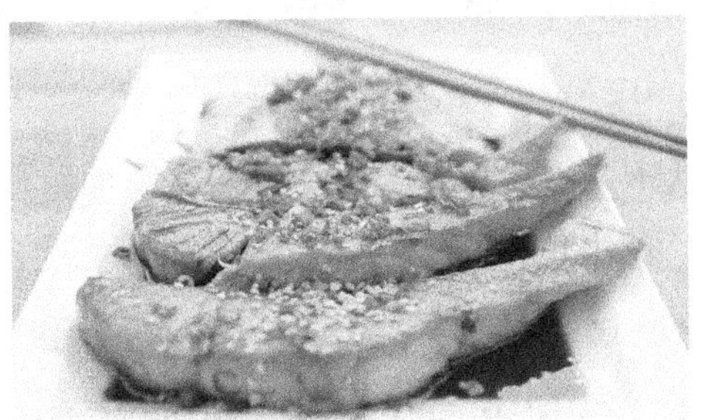

When it comes to healthy protein, there are few more healthy options than fish as it contains several different healthy oils in addition to the right amount of lean protein. This is not the same for farm-raised fish, however, as they are typically much lower in healthier nutrients than their all-natural counterparts. Good choices when it comes to fish includes halibut, Mahi-Mahi, sardines, sole, tuna, snapper, catfish, salmon and anchovies. The same thing goes for shellfish include muscles, oysters, shrimp, crabs, and lobster. Red meat is also a viable alternative assuming the cut is lean in fat and that the animals were raised in an organic and grass-fed environment. Reasonable options in this arena include veal, lamb, venison and beef.

Fats and oils: First and foremost, when it comes to balancing out the fats that you consume each day it is important to balance your intake of omega 3 and omega 6 as you need a balance of both to maintain a healthy lifestyle in the long term. Fish contain plenty of both types of omega fat, though if you are not a fan of fish then fish oil supplements can work just as well.

When it comes to the best monounsaturated or saturated fats the best choices are those that are the most chemically stable as this is a sign that they are good for your health as well. Great choices in this category include things like avocado oil, egg yolks, coconut oil, organic, grass-fed butter and macadamia nuts in moderation.

Carbohydrates: With only a very small percentage of your overall daily intake dedicated to carbohydrates, it is important that you make the amount you can eat as effective as possible. The best way to do this is to focus on vegetables that have the overall lowest amount of carbohydrates as possible so you can maximize the nutritional impact of that portion of your diet. The vegetables that you should avoid at all costs include peppers of all colors, carrots, tomatoes, corn, squash, and peas.

On the other hand, the vegetables that have the lowest overall number of carbs include garlic, kale, cabbage, sprouts, spinach, shallots, olives, radishes, cucumbers, leeks, mushrooms, cauliflower, broccoli, chives, asparagus, dill pickles, and bok choy. If your favorite vegetable didn't make the cut, simply ask yourself if it is starchy, sweet or not green. If you can answer no to all three, then it is probably safe to eat in moderation.

Fats that are healthy for you

Saturated
- ! Lard
- ! Tallow
- ! Chicken fats
- ! Goose fats
- ! Duck fats
- ! Ghee
- ! Coconut oil
- ! Butter
- ! Clarified butter

Monounsaturated

- ! Olive oil
- ! Avocado oil
- ! Macadamia oil

Polyunsaturated

- ! Omega threes that are often found in seafood or fatty fish

Vegetables that do not have starch

Greens

- ! Lettuce
- ! Bok choy
- ! Swiss chard
- ! Chives
- ! Chard
- ! Spinach
- ! Radicchio
- ! Endive

Cruciferous vegetables

- ! Kale (the dark leaf one is the best for you)
- ! Radishes
- ! Kohlrabi

Other

- ! Cucumber
- ! Asparagus
- ! Celery Stalks
- ! Summer squash
- ! Spaghetti squash
- ! Bamboo shoots
- ! Zucchini

Fruit

- ! Avocado

Soy products

Try and stick with non-GMO soy products if you have to eat them. Fermented soy products are good too.

- ! Soy sauce
- ! Natto
- ! Tempeh
- ! Coconut aminos that are paleo friendly
- ! Green soybeans
- ! Black soybeans

Avoid

These are the foods that you are going to want to avoid because they are meats that are factory farmed, food that is processed, and rich in carbohydrates.

Processed foods

- ! Carrageenan
- ! Wheat gluten
- ! Soy products (this is not just for the diet, but your health in general)
- ! Tropical dried fruits
- ! Tropical fruit juices
- ! Tropical fruits
- ! Alcohol
- ! Sweet drinks
- ! Milk
- ! Low-fat products
- ! Zero carb products
- ! Low carb products
- ! Oils or fats that are refined

- ! Artificial sweeteners
- ! Sulfites
- ! BPAs
- ! MSG
- ! Food with carrageenan

Factory farmed fish and pork

- ! Fish with PCBs
- ! Fish inflamed with omega 6
- ! Fish that is high in mercury

Grains

- ! HFCS
- ! Soft drinks
- ! Agave syrup
- ! Sweet pudding
- ! Ice cream
- ! Table sugar
- ! Crackers
- ! Bread
- ! Cookies

- Pizza
- Pasta
- Quinoa
- White potatoes
- Sprouted Grains
- Buckwheat
- Rice
- Amaranth
- Sorghum
- Rice
- Bulgur
- Barley
- Millet
- Oats
- Rye
- Corn
- Wheat
- Wholemeal

Chapter 3:

Keto Tips for Success

Know the equation: The truth is, weight loss comes down to a simple equation of calories in versus calories out. Although there are certain other factors which may play a part, such as your age or any medications you're on, weight loss, in general, comes down to a simple argument of burned energy. If you eat more calories than you burn, you'll gain weight; if you eat fewer calories than you burn, you'll lose weight.

Your body has a certain amount of calories that it burns as a result of your natural biological processes. This is referred to as your basal metabolic rate. This will vary depending on things such as your height, weight, and age. However, these are the calories which you burn without any effort on your end at all!

A lot of people think that you have to be an active

person in order to lose weight. This isn't actually the truth. In order to lose weight, you simply have to eat fewer calories than you burn. As long as you eat less than your metabolic rate, you will lose weight. However, it's worth adding that working out is a major boon to your process of getting healthier. Losing weight is only one aspect of a much bigger spider web of increasing your overall physical health. Working out allows you to maintain the muscle mass that you've already got so that your body doesn't burn it off, and also allows you to tone up as you go.

To find your basal metabolic rate you will want to use one of the following equations:

For men: BMR = 10 x weight (kg) + 6.25 x height (cm) − 5 x age (years) + 5
For women: BMR = 10 x weight (kg) + 6.25 x height (cm) − 5 x age (years) − 161

Avoid trying to lose too much too fast: It's really easy to try to lose more than 2 pounds per week and dial on huge calorie deficits with the idea that you're going to "fight through the pain". However, even 2 pounds per week can really be too much. The body isn't prepared for drastic changes in any way, and this is an easy way to send your body into a "shock" state. It can take a toll on your overall health and can lead to you being far weaker and losing important muscle mass.

What's more is that if you ever find yourself eating less than 1,000 calories per day, you're probably eating too few. For most people, 800 is the starvation threshold. Your body is not made to function on that few calories.

Additionally, if you try to lose a ton of weight all at once, your body is not going to look good. You are going to develop a lot of loose skin and you will not be in proper shape. You may look better than you did when you were fat, but by just practicing proper patience, you can slim down and look good. The only excuse for rapid weight loss is if you're already heavy enough for it to be a major strain on your health, and even then, there's no excuse for eating less than 1,000 calories per day ever. Don't do that. You will hurt yourself.

In the end, I'm sure you've heard that phrase before that weight loss is a marathon and not a sprint. Take your time. If you try to eat too little, you may end up burning out and hardly losing any weight at all. Take it easy on yourself and just try to lose 1 to 1 and a half pounds per week.

Find satisfying substitutes: Take the extra time to seek out substitutes for your favorites. If you find yourself with a particular foodstuff or two that always seems to make you break your diet, consider seeking out healthy substitutes instead. While certain items seem as though they would be impossible to recreate, you will be surprised what the internet can come up with. Do a little digging and you are sure to find an option that will make you forget all about your guilty pleasure.

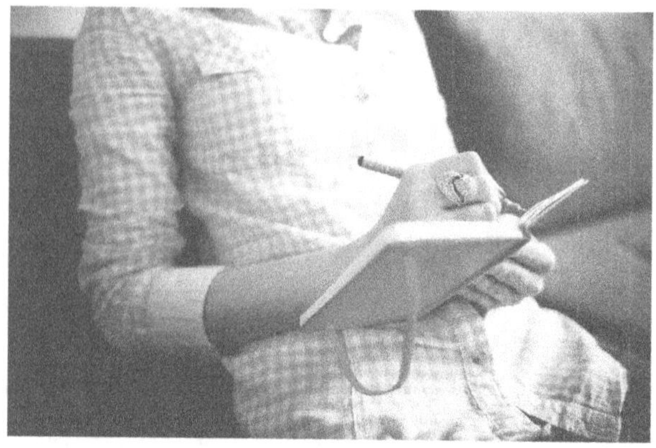

Keep a journal: Although it's not a requirement, you may want to start writing a personal journal or diary regarding your diet. You do not have to be a professional writer to do this.

However, there are two things that you have to do:

>   !   Update your journal regularly (preferably daily)

>   !   Be completely honest with everything that you write in your journal

If you are not that fond of the actual act of writing, then you might want to use a computer or even your mobile phone. Just create a file that you can update easily. The important thing is to have something that you can write on regularly and to be sure that so your writings will be saved and not get won't be lost. These days, there are many free writings apps and software that you can easily download with just a press of a button or a click of a mouse. Of course, it is still recommended that you do it the old-fashioned way: with a notebook and a pen.

Having a journal will allow you to view yourself from a different standpoint, from a perspective that is free from any bias. This is also a good way to see how you can better improve yourself. This is why you have to update your journal regularly and be honest with every record that you write. Your journal will serve as a mirror of yourself.

Since it is your own personal journal, you are free to write everything that you want. Ideally, it should include your reasons for going on a keto diet, your objectives, your thoughts and feelings, your experiences as you go through the diet, and others. In the first few weeks, you might not fully appreciate the value of the journal, but just be more patient. After some time, you will start to appreciate just how helpful it is to have a journal, especially once you notice your progress on the diet.

Don't forget MCT oil: While on the ketogenic diet, the use of high-quality medium chain triglyceride (MCT) oil is crucial in maintaining the state of ketosis. This is because this oil allows those that consume it to eat more carbs/proteins and still maintain a good level of ketosis. You can not only cook with this oil but add it to coffee, tea, green drinks, protein shakes and more!

MCT oil is created with unique fatty acids that are found in palm and coconut oils. They are capable of stabilizing blood sugar levels as they enhance ketone production. This is why MCT is so darn powerful for those on the ketogenic diet! It also has the power to reduce inflammation throughout the body, enhances metabolism as well as cognitive function.

MCT oil is easily digested by the body, which means your body doesn't need to produce more bile to process it. Other fatty acids rely on bile to emulsify them to be absorbed effectively. MCT also has a lower calorie effect than other fatty acids, with only 8.3 calories per gram consumed.

MCT makes ketone levels rise, which allows room for blood sugars to balance out and lower naturally. They are also well-known for their ability to stabilize sugars and help with inflammation and overall brain function. After just one dose of MCT oil, there is a small drop in blood sugar which is caused by the decrease of glucose the liver delivers to the body.

When you consume MCT oil, you are helping your body improve its ability to absorb magnesium and calcium. With MCT, there is a major improvement in nitrogen content overall absorption of proteins, which means your body is more effective in preserving lean muscle.

Don't be afraid to make special requests: For some, the thought of being "that person" makes them squirm. But, at the end of the day, you have a responsibility to take care of yourself and as long as you keep requests respectful and attainable, you should have relatively little pushback. You should prepare yourself for some discomfort, but don't let that interfere with your health goals.

It's pretty standard these days to request burgers at fast food places without the bun; some joints even have these options on the main menu. Nutrition facts are also now readily available at any restaurant making it easier to quickly customize meal choices. You're more likely to get confused or irritated responses from employees for special requests made at fast food restaurants, so try to keep these as simple as possible.

Asking for a burger "protein style" or lettuce wrapped is common enough. Don't give a long list of what you want or don't want; ask for cheese if you want cheese, specify toppings, then just get it dry. You can most likely get a ranch and/or mustard easily enough on the side when you pick up your order. Be prepared for screw-ups on fast food special orders...it's just how it goes.

At sit down restaurants, you will be able to request more sophisticated alterations. It's actually pretty common to ask for no added salt to your meal and most sit-down and family restaurants (chains especially) now have lite or low-carb sections in their menus. Those options make it much easier to get Keto appropriate meals without having to make special requests. Still, it is important to pay attention to additives listed in nutrition facts and sides that come with a meal. A grilled chicken dish is always a good low-carb choice. If it comes with steamed or even sautéed veggies, as long as butter or olive oil is used.

Plan accordingly: Meal planning takes time and cannot happen in an hour. When you plan, shop, and prep as soon as you can, you are not giving yourself a sufficient amount of time to process everything, which can make it more of a stressful experience than it must be. The solution then is to allow yourself ample time to plan meals, especially as a beginner. Set aside 2 to 3 hours per week. Take advantage of the weekend to spread out planning, shopping, and prepping meals. This will allow prepping to feel like a sustainable task that you can do for months to come.

It is also important to not be too ambitious, meal planning should be viewed as a marathon, not a sprint to the finish. You will feel super inspired at the start of your meal prep journey, but once you start to get into the depths of planning, you can become easily overwhelmed. You need to ensure your prep schedule matches your regular schedule so you can sustain it. This is why it is important to create clearly defined goals and assessing your daily routine and schedule; this will help you to find what is realistic for you. Start small and start prepping 2 to 3 nights per week. This will give you the opportunity to figure out what works and what doesn't and allows you to tweak it to your liking.

Avoid temptation: If you are a shopped that gets distracted by grocery store displays, sales, and deals, then you may want to consider purchasing your items online instead. This helps you to avoid aisles that are loaded with temptations that will do nothing but take you off course.

Also, never go shopping at the supermarket when you are hungry. Also, try to do your best not to take your kids. Stores purposely place sugary confections and snacks at children's eye level, knowing it can increase your spending. If you do go shopping with your kids, avoid aisles and shop the perimeter of the store instead. Teach your kids about making good eating choices and how to budget wisely. Children have a secret sixth sense to discover your weak links; firmly say 'no.'

Improve your gut's mobility: A huge challenge the keto dieter must overcome is constipation. This is attributed to an increase of hormones and your blood sugars pulling your body in and out of ketosis. Constipation results from being dehydrated, stress, not enough electrolytes, not eating enough fibrous veggies, etc.

Ensure that you include fermented foods in your keto diet, such as sauerkraut, kefir, coconut water, and kimchi. I highly suggest juicing. I juice my very own fresh green juice in the morning, which helps me to boost my electrolytes and balance my body to maintain my ketosis level. You may also consider supplementing magnesium as well.

Avoid alcohol: While you will naturally want to avoid wine and beer while following the keto diet, all types of alcohol are known to slow the metabolism as it affects the central nervous system. Additionally, when it is consumed along with a meal that is already high in calories it helps to ensure that more of that fat ends up being stored directly in the body as opposed to burned immediately for fuel.

Don't forget vitamin supplements: Especially early on in your new lifestyle, you may find it difficult to naturally acquire all the vitamins and nutrients your body needs to stay healthy. That is why it is extremely important to find a quality multivitamin and take it regularly until, at the very least, you feel comfortable getting what you need from other sources. B12 and vitamin D are two compounds specifically that many people can typically have a hard time acquiring enough of. B12 can be found in specific supplements. Vitamin D can be absorbed from the sun. Spend 30 extra minutes outside every day and you should be able to balance out the difference.

Women shouldn't give up on dairy: Studies show that women who consumed a steady amount of dairy products that were high in fat were able to burn fat almost twice as easily as those who abstained completely. This is the case because calcium works as a sort of switch that tells the female body to up the rate at which fat is burned. What' s more, this occurs only with calcium that comes specifically from dairy products, pills or other sources of calcium just aren't as effective. The goal should be 1,200 mg of calcium each day for the best results.

Eat all the colors of the rainbow: When it comes to vegetables, you should take special care to eat lots of dark, leafy greens as they tend to pack in the most nutrition per ounce. With that being said, however, it is important to mix and match the vegetables you are eating to ensure you are consuming some of every color possible. Different colors equate to different vitamins and nutrients, take advantage of easy access to required nutrients you may not now be getting elsewhere.

Work on your stress levels: Studies show that those with higher overall levels of stress tend to have higher levels of fat in the abdominal region as well. This is caused by the fact that stress releases a hormone known as cortisol which slows your metabolism while at the same time increasing your appetite and telling your body that it is a good time to store as much fat as possible. If you are looking for a good way to get your stress levels moving in the right direction, yoga will help to stimulate the chemical reactions your body needs to start calming down sooner than later.

Chapter 4:

The Importance of Fat Bombs

Once you have made the decision to cut almost all of the carbohydrates from your diet, you'll need to come up with additional ways to feel full and gain energy between meals. This is where fat bombs come in; fat bombs are quick and easy to eat snacks that are typically made from a small number of sweet or savory ingredients as well as seeds, nuts, coconut oil and butter making them almost completely made up of the healthy fats your body is now relying upon.

These concentrated energy snacks will quickly fill you up and prevent you from breaking down during the day and reaching for something that's been processed and packed with carbohydrates. They are a great choice before the gym or when you are struggling to make it from lunch all the way to dinner. Plus, getting the required amount of fat in your diet every day can be more difficult than it first appears. Remember, it is important to always stick to healthy fats otherwise you are just binging on items that have little true nutritional value.

Fat Bomb precautions: Like any other new dietary supplement, when you first begin trying out different fat bomb recipes it is important to do so cautiously at first as you never know how your body might respond. As previously discussed, it's likely that your body hasn't regularly consumed this much healthy fat before, it may take a little while to accept the change. However, if you keep at it you should find that you have adapted to the change relatively quickly. It is important to consume fat bombs in moderation as relying on them too heavily can cause a dependence to form. What this means is that while they can certainly be part of your ketogenic diet plan, then shouldn't be a foundational pillar. Generally speaking one or two per day is a good limit to set.

Create your own: While you will find a variety of fat bomb recipes below to help you get started, creating your own is as simple as finding snacks that are low in carbs and high in fat that will satisfy either a craving for savory or sweet foods. This makes your options in this department extremely malleable as the only true requirements are healthy fats and lots of them. When it comes to creating your own fat bombs, your goal should be items that are about 85 percent fat to keep them as effective as they can be. Another common theme with most fat bomb recipes are a limited number of ingredients, typically with a base of healthy fats, grass-fed butter, coconut oil, and cream cheese are all good places to start. Some additional flavoring in the form of a few extra ingredients should wrap things up most of the time. Keep it simple and you are more likely to discover exciting new flavor combinations.

When it comes to choosing a base fat, the most healthy of the bunch is typically coconut oil as it is the type of fat that is used up the quickest when the body is in ketosis. Many types of fat bombs are chilled or frozen so that they can reach a solid state which means you are going to want to avoid making plans to take most of them with you as well.

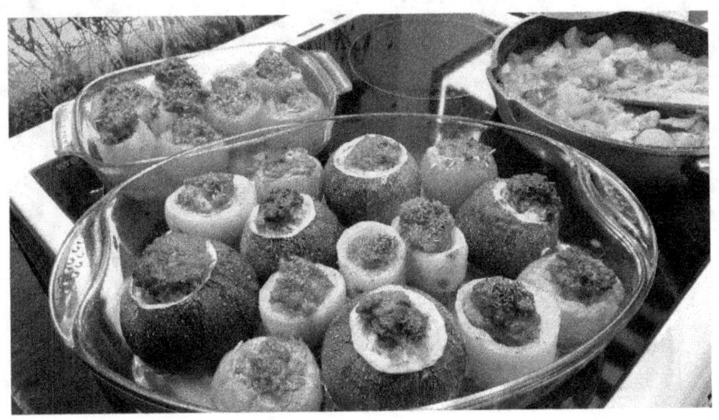

Stuffed Poblano Peppers

Total Prep & Cooking Time: 4 hours and 5 minutes

Yields: 4 Servings

Nutrition stats (one serving)
! Net Carbs: 0.5 grams

- ! Fats: 6.5 grams

- ! Calories: 150

- ! Protein: 17.2 grams

What to Use

- ! Salt (as desired)

- ! Pepper (as desired)

- ! Tomato juice (3 T)

- ! Onion (1 T chopped)

- ! Ground beef (.3 lbs.)

- ! Cauliflower (.3 c chopped fine)

- ! Poblano pepper (1)

What to Do

- ! Slice the poblano pepper in two and remove all of the seeds before setting it aside.

- ! Place the onion and the ground beef in a skillet before placing the skillet on the stove over a burner turned to a high/medium heat and cook for approximately 5 minutes. Stir regularly to ensure the ground beef browns fully.

! Add the results to the poblano halves.

! Add the tomato juice to the slow cooker before placing the stuffed peppers on top.

! Adjust the slow cooker temperature to low and leave it be, covered for about 4 hours.

Brussel sprout dip

Total Prep & Cooking Time: 2 hours 10 minutes
Yields: 4 Servings

Nutrition stats (one serving)
! Net Carbs: 0.2 grams

! Fats: 33 grams

! Calories: 396

! Protein: 13 grams

What to Use
! Salt (as desired)

! Pepper (as desired)

! Parmesan cheese (.25 c grated)

- Mozzarella cheese (.75 c shredded)

- Mayonnaise (.25 c)

- Sour cream (.25 c)

- Cream cheese (4 oz. room temperature)

- Thyme (.5 tsp. chopped)

- Garlic (2 cloves)

- Olive oil (1 T)

- Brussels sprouts (1 lb. quartered, trimmed)

What to Do

- Ensure your oven is heated to 400F.

- Mix together the pepper and salt in a small bowl and the olive oil in another. Dip the brussels sprouts in the oil and then roll them in the second bowl so they are well coated. Place them on the baking sheet in a single layer along with the garlic and cloves.

- Place the baking dish in the oven and let it cook for about 20 minutes, flipping after 10 minutes.

! Place each ingredient into your slow cooker, after squeezing the garlic from its skin and mix well. Adjust the slow cooker temperature to high and leave it be, covered, for about 2 hours.

Chocolate Muffins

Total Prep & Cooking Time: 23 minutes
Yields: 12 Servings

Nutrition stats (one serving)

! Protein: 12 grams

! Net Carbs: 0.7 grams

! Fats: 24 grams

! Calories: 250

What to Use

! Apple cider vinegar (5 ml)

! Coconut oil (25 ml)

! Caramel syrup (50 ml)

! Cocoa powder (5 oz.)

- Golden flaxseed (25 oz.)
- Cinnamon (1 T)
- Baking powder (.5 tsp.)
- Salt (.5 tsp.)
- Slivered almonds (4.5 oz.)

What to Do

- Preheat oven to 350F.
- Mix all dry ingredients (except for the almonds) together in a bowl.
- Mix all wet ingredients together in a bowl.
- Combine the dry and wet ingredients together.
- Pour mixture into muffin liners.
- Sprinkle almond slivers on top of each muffin.
- Bake muffins for 15 minutes.

Tiramisu

Total Prep & Cooking Time: 45 minutes
Yields: 4 Servings

Nutrition stats (one serving)

- ! Protein: 16.2 grams
- ! Net Carbs: 0.8 grams
- ! Fats: 25 grams
- ! Calories: 147

What to Use - Sponge Cake Base

- Egg whites (6)
- Dymatise Nutrition Elite egg protein (35 grams)
- Cream of tartar (.25 tsp.)
- Coconut flour (15 grams)

What to Use - (Faux) Mascarpone Layer

- Fat-free quark (250 grams)
- Vanilla-flavored whey protein (28 grams)

What to Use – Everything Else

- Espresso (60 ml)
- Raw cocoa powder (1 tsp.)

What to Do

- Separate the egg yolks from the egg whites.

- Whip the egg whites together with the cream of tartar until it stiffens and peaks.

- In a separate mixing bowl, mix the coconut flour and protein powder together. Fold in gently to mix together with the egg white and cream of tartar mixture.

- Pour the sponge cake batter into a baking paper-lined pan.

- Bake between 20 and 30 minutes until browned and almost hard.

- Poke holes into the sponge cake. Pour coffee on it.

- Use a cake pan that is half the size of the one used for baking the cake.

- Cut the sponge cake down the middle, making two equal halves.

- Cut the sponge cake down the middle of each half, making four equal pieces.

- In a bowl, mix the whey protein and the quark.

- Put the first cake layer in the pan and

spread one-quarter of the quark mixture on top. Dust the top with cocoa powder.

- Repeat the layering of the cake, the quark mixture and the cocoa powder for the other layers.

- Refrigerate overnight.

Nougat Treats

Total Prep & Cooking Time: 30 minutes
Yields: 40 Servings

Nutrition stats (one serving)

! Protein: 1.2 grams

! Net Carbs: 0.2 grams

! Fats: 26 grams

! Calories: 76

What to Use

- Vanilla (1 tsp)

- Cocoa powder (1 T)

- Peanut butter (8 T)

- Coconut milk (14 oz.)
- Coconut oil (.5 c divided)
- Dark chocolate (7.5 oz)

What to Do

- Melt half of the chocolate and mix in two T of the coconut oil.

- Pour this into a parchment-lined a greased square baking dish, and place in the fridge to harden.

- Add the solid part of the coconut milk to a pot and allow it to come to a simmer.

- Add in .25 cup coconut oil, vanilla, cocoa powder, and nut butter. Mix together until smooth. If it starts to split, use an electric mixer to bring it together.

- Take the mixture off the heat and pour into the baking dish. Refrigerate again until firm. Melt the rest of the chocolate just like in step one.

- Spread this over top of the chilled nougat and refrigerate again.

- Slice into 40 pieces and keep in a storage container in the fridge.

Granola

Total Prep & Cooking Time: 40 minutes

Yields: 12 Servings

Nutrition stats (one serving)

- ! Protein: 7.9 grams
- ! Net Carbs: 0.4 grams
- ! Fats: 31.6 grams
- ! Calories: 337

What to Use

- ! Swerve (.5c)
- ! Salt (1 tsp.)
- ! Pumpkin seeds (1 c)
- ! Raw almonds (.5c)
- ! Raw walnuts (.5c)
- ! Vanilla extract (1 tsp.)
- ! Raw pecans (.5c)

- ! Raw hazelnuts (.5c)
- ! Raw sunflower seeds (1 c)
- ! Vanilla Stevia (1 tsp)
- ! Ground cinnamon (1 tsp)
- ! Unsweetened shredded coconut (1 c)
- ! Coconut oil (.3 c)

What to Do

- ! Set the cooker to sauté then add the coconut oil and melt. When melted, add the vanilla extract and Stevia. Stir well before adding coconut, seeds, and nuts. Stir mixture well to coat all ingredients.
- ! In bowl whisk salt, cinnamon, and swerve then sprinkle with seeds and nuts.
- ! Close and seal the lid. Set on slow cook on low for two hours and stir every 30 minutes.
- ! When done, quick release the pressure. Spread onto a baking pan to cool and store in an airtight container.

Eggs in a Cup

Total Prep & Cooking Time: 10 minutes

Yields: 4 Servings

Nutrition stats (one serving)

- ! Protein: 9 grams
- ! Net Carbs: 0.3 grams
- ! Fats: 29 grams
- ! Calories: 115

What to Use

- ! Salt (as desired)
- ! Pepper (as desired)
- ! Heavy cream (.25 c)
- ! Cilantro (2 T)
- ! Cheddar cheese (1 c)
- ! Shredded cheese (.5c)
- ! Diced veggies (1 c)
- ! Eggs (4 large)

What to Do

- ! Combine the cilantro, pepper, salt, half & half, cheese, veggies, and eggs and divide into four-pint jars. Loosely place on lids.
- ! Add two cups water to the pot and trivet. Set the jars. Lock the lid and set the cooker on high for five minutes. Once done, release the pressure.
- ! Add other cheese and broil for a few minutes.

Spiced Bacon Deviled Eggs

Total Prep & Cooking Time: 15 minutes
Yields: 3 Servings

Nutrition stats (one serving)

- ! Protein: 12.6 grams
- ! Net Carbs: 0.8 grams
- ! Fats: 28 grams
- ! Calories: 315

What to Use

- Rosemary (.5tsp)
- Cayenne (.25 tsp)
- Dijon (1 tsp)
- Bacon fat (1 T)
- Bacon (2 slices)
- Mayo (.25 c)
- Eggs (5 hardboiled)

What to Do

- Crumble up your cooked bacon and slice the eggs in half. Remove the yolks into a bowl. Mix half of the rosemary, the bacon fat, cayenne, Dijon, and mayo.
- Place some pieces of bacon into the bottom of each egg. Pipe the yolk mixture in each of the eggs and top with the rest of the bacon and rosemary.

Pizza Chips

Total Prep & Cooking Time: 25 minutes

Yields: 21Servings

Nutrition stats (one serving)

- ! Protein: 3 grams

- ! Net Carbs: 0.1 grams

- ! Fats: 24 grams

- ! Calories: 62

What to Use

- ! Mozzarella (5.25 oz shredded)

- ! Pepperoni (6 oz sliced)

What to Do

- ! Your oven should be placed on 400F. Arrange the pepperoni in batches of four, layer on each other, onto some cookie sheets. Place this in the oven for about five minutes.

- ! Sprinkle the cheese on each of them and bake for three more minutes.

- Set the chips on paper towels to soak up the grease and enjoy.

Cheese and Bacon Balls

Nutrition stats (one serving)

- Protein: 8.1 grams
- Net Carbs: 1.1 grams
- Fats: 28 grams
- Calories: 284

What to Use

- Bacon (5.3 oz)
- Butter (1 T)
- Cream cheese (5.3 oz)
- Cheddar cheese (5.3 oz)
- Butter (2 oz room temp)

What to Do

- Melt one T butter in skillet fry bacon until crispy.
- Crumble into small pieces and put in a bowl.

! In a large bowl add bacon grease and remaining ingredients. Mix well using either an electric mixer or by hand.

! Put in refrigerator for 15 minutes to harden.

! Make 24 walnut-sized balls. Roll into crumbled bacon.

Stuffed Mini Peppers

Total Prep & Cooking Time: 40 minutes
Yields: 6 Servings

Nutrition stats (one serving)

! Protein: 19.6 grams

! Net Carbs: 0.6 grams

! Fats: 30 grams

! Calories: 304

What to Use

! Fresh thyme (1 T)

! Olive oil (2 T)

! Mild chipotle paste (.5 T)

! Chorizo (30 grams dried, sliced)

! Cream cheese (8 oz)

! Mini bell peppers (8 oz)

What to Do

! Cut the pepper in half lengthwise and remove the core.

! Chop herbs and sausage very fine.

! Mix oil, spices, and cheese in a small bowl. Add herbs and sausage. Mix well.

! Spread mixture into each of the bell pepper halves. Serve.

Chapter 5:

Sample Meal Plan

What follows is a seven-day meal plan designed to help you get started on your ketogenic journey. Each meal is specially chosen to be as low in carbohydrates as possible to ensure that at no point do you go over 15 net grams of carbs per day. You will want to be careful when it comes to adding in fat bombs to these early meals unless you know for a fact you have some extra carbs left in your day.

Day 1

Breakfast Mozzanormal Tacos

Total Prep & Cooking Time: 40 minutes

Yields: 6 Servings

Nutrition stats (one serving)

- Protein: 26 grams
- Net Carbs: 3 grams
- Fats: 36 grams
- Calories: 450

What to Use

- Eggs (8)
- Bacon (.5 lbs.)
- Avocado (1)
- Butter (3 T)
- Mozzarella cheese (2 c shredded)
- .25

What to Do

! You will first need to prepare the bacon. You can cook this in a pan and drain the excess fat, or you can place the bacon on tinfoil and cook it in the oven. In either case, you want the bacon to come out crispy, browned and maybe slightly chard – this is for the texture of crispiness for the tacos.

! Next, you need to prepare your shells using the shredded mozzarella. Take a medium size skillet and place it over medium heat. Take around .3 a c of shredded cheese and place it in the pan in the shape of a pancake. It will take around 3 minutes for the mozzarella to cook together to form the shell. You will know it is ready when the edges of the cheese start to brown.

! After you have removed the mozzarella from the pan, you will need to drape it over a spoon or spatula that is stretched across a bowl (think about it as hanging clothes on a line to dry). The idea here is to get the cheese while it's still hot and malleable to form a taco shell. You will have 1-2 minutes before the cheese hardens and the shape is permanent. Repeat steps 2 and 3 for each taco shell.

! Cook scrambled eggs, using the same skillet as the mozzarella for convenience.

! Cut your avocado into six slices. Also, slice up your bacon into little strips to fit in the tacos.

! Place the scrambled eggs in each taco shell, followed by the bacon and then avocado. Serve immediately.

Lunch: Chicken and broccoli zucchini boats

Total Prep & Cooking Time: 25 minutes

Yields: 4 Servings

Nutrition stats (one serving)

- ! Protein: 30 grams

- ! Net Carbs: 3.5 grams

- ! Fats: 34 grams

- ! Calories: 476

What to Use

- ! Chicken (6 oz. shredded)

- ! Butter (2 T)

- ! Zucchini (2 hollowed-out)

- ! Cheddar cheese (3 oz. shredded)

- ! Green onion (1 stalk)

- ! Broccoli (1 c)

- ! Sour cream (2 T)

What to Do

- ! Preset the oven to 400F.

- ! Slice the zucchini lengthwise and scoop most of the insides until you have a shell of approximately .5 to 1 cm. thick.

- ! Melt 1 T of the butter into each boat, flavor with a dash of pepper and salt if you wish and bake them for around twenty minutes.

- ! Shred the chicken, cut the broccoli florets into small pieces, and measure out six oz. of cheese. Mix with the sour cream.

- ! Remove the zucchini shells when done and add the mixture.

- ! Sprinkle each of them with the remainder of the cheese.

- ! Bake for another ten or fifteen minutes until the cheese is browned and melted.

- ! Use a bit of mayo, sour cream, or chopped onion as a garnish.

Dinner: Italian Mushroom Frittata

Total Prep & Cooking Time: 55 minutes

Yields: 2 Servings

Nutrition stats (one serving)

- Protein: 14 grams
- Net Carbs: 4 grams
- Fats: 36 grams
- Calories: 450

What to Use

- Mayonnaise (.5 c)
- Eggs (5)
- Scallions (3 chopped)
- Butter (1.5 oz. divided)
- Mushrooms (.5 lb.)
- Parsley (.5 T)
- Mozzarella cheese (.25 lb. shredded)
- Salt (as desired)
- Pepper (as desired)

What to Do

- Preheat your oven to 350F.
- Cut the mushrooms for the omelet, making the pieces as small or large as you would like. Cook the mushrooms over medium heat in a skillet, using butter to sauté.
- Add the cooked mushrooms, chopped scallions, and parsley to a medium size mixing bowl. Add salt and pepper to taste.
- In a separate mixing medium size mixing bowl, stir together the eggs, mayonnaise, and cheese.
- Using a large baking tray, pour the cooked mushroom mix along with the egg mix. Stir in the baking tray but don't worry about how well mixed all of these ingredients are.
- Bake in the oven for 30-40 minutes, or until the eggs are cooked to a golden brown color.
- Let cool 5 minutes and serve.

Day 2

Breakfast: Ketogenic Buttered Eggs

Total Prep & Cooking Time: 10 minutes

Yields: 1 Serving

Nutrition stats (one serving)
- Protein: 13 grams
- Net Carbs: 2 grams
- Fats: 27 grams
- Calories: 311

What to Use
- ! Eggs (3)
- ! Butter (2 T)
- ! Garlic (2 cloves)
- ! Coconut oil (1 T)
- ! Cumin (.5 tsp ground)
- ! Sea salt (.5 tsp)
- ! Cayenne (.5 tsp ground)

! Parsley (.3 c)

! Cilantro (.3 c)

! Thyme (1 tsp)

What to Do

! Heat butter and coconut oil in a skillet.

! Add garlic cloves and cook for three minutes.

! Add the thyme and cook for 30 seconds.

! Next, add parsley and cilantro and cook for three minutes.

! Last, add eggs into the skillet and cook for 4-6 minutes. If you enjoy your eggs runnier, only cook for 3-4 minutes.

! If you are looking for added protein, add in breakfast sausage for extra flavor.

Lunch: Egg and Pork Quiche

Total Prep & Cooking Time: 35 minutes

Yields: 2 Servings

Nutrition stats (one serving)

- Protein: 33 grams
- Net Carbs: 3 grams
- Fats: 34 grams
- Calories: 477

What to Use

! Ketogenic Pie Crust (1)

! Eggs (4 large)

! Pork loin (12 oz.)

! Cheddar cheese (.5 c)

! Cream cheese (1 c)

! Garlic (2 cloves)

! Red onion (1)

! Bacon (5 slices)

! Ghee (1 T)

! Black pepper (as desired)

! Pink Himalayan salt (as desired)

! Chives (.5 c chopped)

What to Do

! Place your ghee into a pan then cook the onion and garlic for five minutes. Once it is done, throw in the bacon and cook for another five minutes.

! When this is cooked through, add your pork loin in and cook until it is browned on both sides.

! As you cook these, you will want to preheat your oven to 400F.

! In a bowl, go ahead and mix your seasonings with the eggs and cream cheese. When well blended, grate cheddar cheese over the top and combine.

! For extra flavor, add in some spring onion or chives. Be sure to mix the eggs well.

! First, place your pork and bacon into your ketogenic pie crust. Once it is spread evenly, you can pour the egg mixture on top.

! Finally, cook the pie in the oven for 25

minutes.

Dinner: Ham and apple flatbread

Total Prep & Cooking Time: 40 minutes
Yields: 8 Servings

Nutrition stats (one serving)
- Protein: 16 grams
- Net Carbs: 2.5 grams
- Fats: 20 grams
- Calories: 255

What to Use - Crust
- ! Almond flour (.75 c)
- ! Mozzarella cheese (2 c grated)
- ! Cream cheese (2 T)
- ! Thyme (1 pinch dried)
- ! Sea salt (.5 tsp.)

What to Use - Topping
- ! Ham (4 oz. sliced)
- ! Red onion (.5 small)
- ! Mexican cheese (1 c grated)

- ! Apple (.25)
- ! Thyme (1 pinch dried)

What to Do

- ! Remove the core and seeds from the apples. You can leave them unpeeled but will need to use a vegetable peeler to make the thin slices.
- ! Preset the oven to 425F.
- ! Cut two pieces of parchment paper to fit into a 12-inch pizza pan (approximately two inches larger than the pan).
- ! Use the high heat setting. Place a double boiler (water in the bottom pan), and bring the water to boiling, place the heat setting to low.
- ! Add the cream cheese, mozzarella cheese, salt, thyme, and almond flour to the top of the double boiler—stirring constantly.
- ! When the cheese mixture resembles dough, place it on one of the pieces of parchment—and knead the dough until totally mixed.
- ! Roll the dough into a ball—placing it on

the center of the paper—place the second piece of paper over the top and roll with a rolling pin (or a large glass).

! Place the dough onto the pizza pan (leaving the paper connected).

! Poke several holes in the dough and put into the preheated oven for approximately six to eight minutes.

! When browned, remove it and lower the setting of the oven to 350F.

! Arrange the cheese, apple slices, onion slices, and ham pieces.

! Top off with the remainder (.75 c) of cheese.

! Flavor with the ground pepper, salt, and thyme.

! Place in the oven and bake until the cheese melted and the crust is to the desired brown.

! Slide it from the parchment paper and cool two or three minutes before cutting.

! Tip: If you do not own a double boiler; you can substitute with a mixing dish over a pot of boiling water as a substitute.

__Day 3__

Breakfast: Broccoli Frittata

Total Prep & Cooking Time: 25 minutes

Yields: 2 Servings

Nutrition stats (one serving)

- Protein: 17 grams
- Net Carbs: 1.8 grams
- Fats: 22 grams
- Calories: 275

What to Use

- ! Bell pepper (.5)
- ! Sausage (1 lb. ground)
- ! Broccoli (1.5 c)
- ! Eggs (7 beaten)
- ! Olives (.25 c. sliced)
- ! Garlic (1 clove minced)
- ! Salt (.5 tsp.)

What to Do

- ! Turn on the oven so that it can warm up to 350F. In the meantime, bring out a skillet and use it to brown up the sausage.

- ! While the sausage is cooking, bring out the food processor and pulse together the bell pepper, garlic, and broccoli so they become small pieces.

- ! Add the bell pepper, broccoli, and salt to the sausage once it is browned. Add the eggs next and let everything cook for 5 minutes so the egg starts to set, making sure not to stir.

- ! Sprinkle your olives on top before taking the skillet off the heat and into the oven for another 10 minutes. Once the egg is set you can take it out of the oven and serve right away.

Lunch: Keto Burger

Total Prep & Cooking Time: 18 minutes

Yields: 2 Servings

Nutrition stats (one serving)

- Protein: 25 grams
- Net Carbs: 4 grams
- Fats: 34 grams
- Calories: 405

What to Use

! Basil (.5 tsp.)

! Cayenne (.25 tsp.)

! Crushed red pepper (.5 tsp.)

! Salt (.5 tsp.)

! Lettuce (2 large leaves)

! Butter (2 T)

! Egg (1 large)

! Sriracha (1 T)

! Onion (.25)

! Plum tomato (.5)

! Mayo (1 T)

! Pickled jalapenos (1 T, sliced)

! Bacon (1 strip)

! Ground beef (.5 lb.)

! Bacon (1 strip)

What to Do

! Knead mean for about three minutes.

! Chop bacon, jalapeno, tomato, and onion into fine pieces. (shown below)

! Knead in mayo, sriracha, egg, and chopped ingredients, and spices into the meat.

! Separate meat into four even pieces and flatten them (not thinly, just press on the tops to create a flat surface). Place a T of butter on top of two of the meat pieces. Take the pieces that do not have butter of them and set them on top of the buttered ones (basically creating a butter and meat sandwich). Seal the sides together, concealing the butter within.

! Throw the patties on the grill (or in a pan) for about 5 minutes on each side. Caramelize some onions if you want too!

! Prepare large leaves of lettuce by spreading some mayo onto them. Once patties are finished, place them on one half of the lettuce, add your desired burger toppings, and fold the other half over of the lettuce leaf over the patty.

! Burger time!

Dinner: Spicy Chicken Casserole

Total Prep & Cooking Time: 30 minutes
Yields: 6 Servings

Nutrition stats (one serving)
- Protein: 35 grams
- Net Carbs: 2.5 grams
- Fats: 36 grams
- Calories: 436

What to Use
! Pepper (as desired)

! Salt (as desired)

! Chili seasoning (1.5 tsp)

! Cream cheese (4 oz.)

! Chicken thighs (1.75 lbs.)

- ! Tomatoes and green chilies (1 c)
- ! Jalapeno pepper (1)
- ! Cauliflower (1 pkg.)
- ! Sour cream (.25 c.)
- ! Olive oil (2 tsp)
- ! Cheddar cheese (4 oz.)
- ! Parmesan cheese (3 tsp)

What to Do

- ! Make sure that your oven gets to 375F. Chop the chicken into small pieces and then season it with chili seasoning, pepper, salt.
- ! Bring out a skillet and cook the chicken so that all of the sides are browned. Add in .75 of the cheddar cheese, the sour cream, and the cream cheese. Stir well until the cheese melts.
- ! Add in the tomatoes with the green chilies and then pour this into a casserole dish.
- ! Microwave the cauliflower so that it cooks through. Put into a bowl and add in the

cheese. Use an immersion blender and then blend this into a mashed potato mixture. Season with pepper and salt.

!   Cut the jalapeno with chunks. Spread the cauliflower mixture on top of the chicken mixture and top with the jalapeno chunks. Place into the oven and bake for 15 minutes. Slice up and serve.

Day 4

Breakfast: Keto Breakfast

Total Prep & Cooking Time: 15 minutes

Yields: 1 Serving

Nutrition stats (one serving)

- Protein: 19.5 grams
- Net Carbs: 3.6 grams
- Fats: 41.3 grams
- Calories: 275

What to Use

! Ghee (1 T)

! Avocado (.5)

! Portobello mushrooms (2)

! Bacon slices (5)

! Egg (1)

What to Do

! To start, pan roast the mushrooms and

heat up half your ghee and cook these until they become tender.

! Cook the bacon and egg as well, either separately or in the same pan.

! Serve with the avocado and enjoy.

Lunch: Avocado Stuffed with Salmon

Total Prep & Cooking Time: 30 minutes

Yields: 2 Servings

Nutrition stats (one serving)

- Protein: 27 grams
- Net Carbs: 2.4 grams
- Fats: 34.6 grams
- Calories: 300

What to Use

! Dill (2 T)

! Ghee (1 T)

! Pepper (as desired)

! Salt (as desired)

- ! Lemon juice (2 T)
- ! Sour cream (.25 c)
- ! Chopped white onion (1)
- ! Salmon fillets (2)
- ! Avocado (2 medium)

What to Do

- ! Turn your oven to heat up to 400F. Take out some parchment paper and place on a baking tray along with the salmon. Season with the lemon juice, pepper, olive oil, and salt.
- ! Let everything bake inside the oven for 25 minutes. Take out when it is done.
- ! Once the fish cools down, use a fork to shred it up, getting rid of the skin, and mix it with the onion, dill, and sour cream.
- ! Scoop out the avocado, leaving just a bit of the flesh and chop up the rest so you can mix with the salmon.
- ! Fill your avocados with the salmon and top with the lemon juice before serving.

Dinner: Keto Chili

Total Prep & Cooking Time: 140 minutes

Yields: 6 Servings

Nutrition stats (one serving)

- Protein: 22 grams
- Net Carbs: 3.4 grams
- Fats: 26.5 grams
- Calories: 412

What to Use

! Garlic (6 cloves)

! Green bell pepper (1)

! Beef (2 lbs.)

! Pepper (as desired)

! Olive oil (2 tsp)

! Chili powder (1.5 tsp)

! Tomatoes (1 can dice)

! Cumin (3 tsp)

What to Do

- ! Form the beef into patties. Heat a little of the oil into a soup pot before adding the black pepper into it.

- ! Next, take the bell peppers and sauté them in the oil in the soup pot for 7 minutes before taking the pot from the heat.

- ! Gently add in the garlic for a few minutes. Turn your grill on before placing the beef patties on it and allowing the meat to cook so they become medium rare.

- ! At this time, you can turn back on the heat and place the soup pot back on the stove before adding the garlic, oil, and pepper into the pot, making sure to break up the patties so they are small pieces before adding.

- ! Finally, add the tomatoes to the mixture, making sure to mash them up well before adding some water so that the ingredients become covered. Allow the whole chili to simmer for a minimum of two hours and then enjoy.

<u>Day 5</u>

Breakfast: High Fiber Keto Cacao Cereal

Total Prep & Cooking Time: 70 minutes

Yields: 1 Serving

Nutrition stats (one serving)

- Protein: 9 grams
- Net Carbs: 2 grams
- Fats: 15 grams
- Calories: 254

What to Use

- Chia Seeds (.5 c)
- Hemp Hearts (4 T)
- Coconut Oil (2 T)
- Raw Cacao Nibs (2 T)
- Organic Sugar-Free Vanilla Extract (1 T)
- Swerve (1 T)
- Fine Psyllium Powder (1 T)
- Water (1 c)

What to Do

- ! Ensure your oven is preheated to 285F.
- ! In a large mixing bowl, cover chia seeds with water, stir once and let sit.
- ! After 5 minutes, add fine psyllium powder, swerve, vanilla extract, coconut oil, and hemp hearts into the bowl with chia seeds. Blend until ingredients are thoroughly mixed and chia seeds start to gel.
- ! Add cacao nibs to the bowl and stir them into the dough.
- ! Place two large pieces of wax paper down. Turn dough out onto wax paper and roll until dough is about 11 x 14 inches across.
- ! Take hands to roll dough into cylinder and place on parchment paper with the shiny side up.
- ! Flatten dough with fingers before you place another piece of parchment paper over it. Flatten until it is .25 inches thick.
- ! Bake 15 minutes. The dough should dry

significantly and be almost completely dry after 15 minutes.

! Remove cookie sheet and carefully flip dough over, removing the parchment paper that will now be on the top side. Cook for an additional 15-25 minutes, until t h e dough is completely dry. Check frequently after 15 minutes to ensure cereal doesn't burn.

! Remove cereal from oven and let cool to at least room temperature before breaking up into smaller chunks to with cream or coconut milk. The remainder can successfully be stored someplace airtight for as many as 3 days.

Lunch: Keto Pasty

Total Prep & Cooking Time: 20 minutes

Yields: 1 Serving

Nutrition stats (one serving)

- Protein: 17 grams

- Net Carbs: 2.1 grams
- Fats: 29.3 grams
- Calories: 375

What to Use - Bread

! Baking powder (.5 tsp.)

! Psyllium husk (.5 T powder)

! Salt (1 pinch)

! Cream cheese (4 oz.)

! Eggs (3)

What to Use - Filling

! Cheese (shredded 4 oz.)

! Garlic (.5 cloves minced)

! Lemon juice (.5 tsp.)

! Olive oil (1 can)

! Dill pickles (.25 c chopped)

! Celery (1 stalk)

! Sour cream (.3 c)

What to Do - Bread

! Start by making sure your oven is heated

to 300F.

! Separate the eggs from their yolks and save both in separate bowls.

! Add salt to the whites and whisk well.

! Add the cream cheese to the yolks and mix well before adding in the baking powder and psyllium.

! Combine the two bowls and mix well before adding the results to a baking sheet so that it will form eight slices.

! Bake in the center of the oven for 25 minutes

What to Do - Filling

! Start by making sure your oven is heated to 350F.

! Combine all of the filling ingredients, minus the cheese, together in a bowl and mix well.

! Place two slices of bread onto a lined baking sheet and top with filling and finish with cheese.

! Bake 15 minutes.

Dinner: Keto Casserole

Total Prep & Cooking Time: 40 minutes

Yields: 2 Servings

Nutrition stats (one serving)

- Protein: 14 grams
- Net Carbs: 3 grams
- Fats: 25 grams
- Calories: 360

What to Use

! Caraway seeds (0.5 tsp.)

! Pickle brine (2 T)

! Low-sugar ketchup (.5 c)

! Cream cheese (8 oz)

! mayonnaise (.5 c)

! Swiss cheese (2 c shredded)

! Sauerkraut (1 can drained)

! Corned beef (.5 lbs. diced)

What to Do

- ! Ensure that your oven has been preheated to 350F.
- ! Place a medium saucepan on the stove top and warm it over low heat. Melt together the mayonnaise, ketchup, and cream cheese.
- ! Following the melting process, add 1.5 c of shredded swiss cheese, the drained sauerkraut, and corned beef. Mix together all of the ingredients until they are incorporated and the cheese has melted.
- ! Before you remove the pan from the stove top, add the pickle brine or a pinch of garlic salt, a tsp. of vinegar, and a T of salt if you do not have pickle brine available.
- ! Prepare a dish by greasing it and pour the results into it carefully. Top it all off with the remaining swiss cheese and garnish with caraway seeds.
- ! Bake the casserole for about 20 minutes, or until mixture starts bubbling and

cheese melts.

Day 6

Breakfast: Steak and eggs with avocado

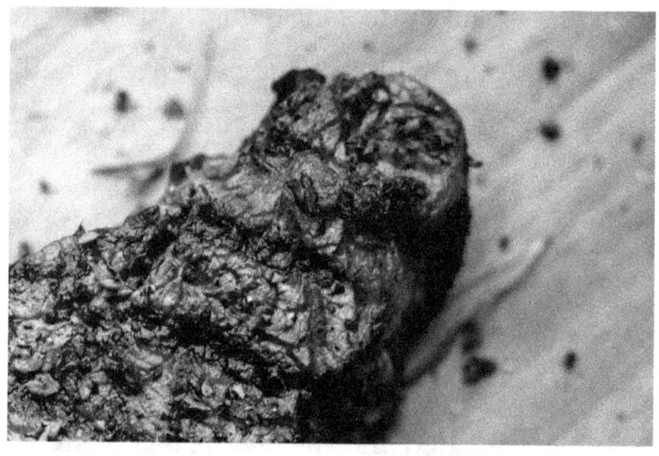

Total Prep & Cooking Time: 15 minutes

Yields: 1 Serving

Nutrition stats (one serving)

- Protein: 44 grams

- Net Carbs: 3 grams

- Fats: 36 grams

- Calories: 379

What to Use

! Salt (as desired)

! Pepper (as desired)

! Avocado (.25 sliced)

! Sirloin steak (4 oz.)

! Eggs (3 large)

! Butter (1 T)

What to Do

! Melt the T of butter in a pan and fry all 3 eggs to the desired doneness. Season the eggs with salt and pepper.

! In a different pan, cook the sirloin steak to your preferred taste and slice it into thin strips. Season the steak with salt and pepper.

! Sever your prepared steak and eggs with slices of avocado.

! Enjoy!

Lunch: Keto Pizza

Total Prep & Cooking Time: 20 minutes

Yields: 2 Servings

Nutrition stats (one serving)

- Protein: 17 grams
- Net Carbs: 1.8 grams
- Fats: 22 grams
- Calories: 275

What to Use - Base

! Oregano (1 tsp.)

! Vegetable oil (7 tsp.)

! Garlic (1 tsp. minced)

! Egg (1 large)

! Parmesan (32 g. grated)

! Mozzarella (1.25 c. grated)

! Cauliflower (1 c)

What to Use - Sauce

! Italian pasta sauce (250 g.)

! Vegetable oil (7 tsp)

! Basil leaves (as desired)

! Garlic (1 tsp. minced)

! Oregano (1 tsp)

! Tomato puree (1 tsp.)

What to Use - Topping

! Mozzarella (1 handful grated)

! Fresh mozzarella (1 small ball)

! Other toppings (as desired)

What to Do

! Grate up the cauliflower until it looks like fine grains of rice. Place this into the microwave for about four minutes and then strain the cauliflower to get rid of the moisture.

! Place the egg, cheese, and seasoning into a big mixing bowl and mix together to make the dough for the pizza. Form this into a base using a pizza pan.

! Turn on the oven to 350F and bake this dough for about 10 minutes.

! While that is baking, it is time to mix the ingredients for the sauce together. When the crust is done, you can spread this sauce all over the crust.

Dinner: Sesame chicken

Nutrition stats (one serving)

- Protein: 45 grams
- Net Carbs: 4 grams
- Fats: 36 grams
- Calories: 275

What to Use

! Broccoli (.75 c, cut bite size)

! Xanthan gum (.25 tsp.)

! Sesame seeds (2 T)

! Garlic (1 clove)

! Ginger (1 cm cube)

! Vinegar (1 T)

! Brown sugar alternative (2 T)

! Soy sauce (2 T)

! Toasted sesame seed oil (2 T)

! Arrowroot powder or cornstarch (1 T)

! Chicken thighs (1lb. cut into bite sized pieces)

! Egg (1 large)

! Salt (as desired)

! Pepper (as desired)

! Chives (as desired)

What to Do

! First, make the batter by combining the egg with a T of arrowroot powder (or cornstarch). Whisk well.

! Place chicken pieces in batter. Be sure to coat all sides of chicken pieces with the batter.

! Heat one T of sesame oil, in a large pan. Add chicken pieces to hot oil and fry. Be gentle when flipping the chicken, you want to keep the batter from falling off. It should take about 10 minutes for them to cook fully.

! Next, make the sesame sauce. In a small bowl, combine soy sauce, brown sugar alternative, vinegar, ginger, garlic, sesame seeds, and the remaining T of toasted sesame seed oil. Whisk very well.

! Once the chicken is fully cooked, add broccoli and the sesame sauce to the pan and cook for an additional 5 minutes.

! Spoon desired amount into a bowl, top it off with some chopped chives, and relish in some fine dining at home!

<u>Day 7</u>

Breakfast: Brownie Muffins

Total Prep & Cooking Time: 25 minutes

Yields: 6 Servings

Nutrition stats (one serving)

- Protein: 7 grams
- Net Carbs: 3.2 grams
- Fats: 13.4 grams
- Calories: 183

What to Use

- Salt (.5 tsp)
- Flaxseed meal (1 c)
- Cocoa powder (.25 c)
- Baking powder (.5 T)
- Cinnamon (1 T)
- Coconut oil (2 T)
- Egg (1 large)
- Sugar-free caramel syrup (.25 c)

! Vanilla extract (1 tsp.)

! Pumpkin puree (.5 c)

! Slivered almonds (.25 c)

! Apple cider vinegar (1 tsp.)

What to Do

! Heat the oven temperature at 350F.

! In a deep mixing bowl—combine all of the ingredients—mixing well.

! Use six paper liners in the muffin tin and add .25 c of the batter to each one.

! Sprinkle several almonds on the tops, pressing gently.

! Bake approximately fifteen minutes. It is done when the top is set.

Lunch: Tuna Cheese Melt

Total Prep & Cooking Time: 25 minutes

Yields: 1 Serving

Nutrition stats (one serving)

- Protein: 19 grams
- Net Carbs: 4.1 grams
- Fats: 26.3 grams
- Calories: 415

What to Use

! Oopsie bread (2 pieces)

What to Use - Salad

! Celery stalks (1 to 2)

! Sour cream or mayonnaise (.3 T)

! Tuna in olive oil (1 can)

! Dill pickles (4 T chopped)

! Lemon juice (.5 tsp.)

! Pepper (as desired)

! Salt (as desired)

! Garlic (.5 clove minced)

What to Use - Toppings

! Paprika powder (1 pinch)

! Cheese (3.5 oz. shredded)

- ! Olive oil (1 T)
- ! Leafy greens (.3 lbs.)

What to Use – Oopsie Bread

- ! Eggs (3)
- ! Salt (1 pinch)
- ! Cream cheese (4.25 oz.)
- ! Baking powder (5 tsp)
- ! Psyllium husk powder (.5 T ground)

What to Do

- ! Preheat the oven to 350F. Put parchment paper onto a cookie sheet.
- ! Blend all of the salad ingredients.
- ! Place the bread slices on the prepared sheet, spread the tuna, and sprinkle the cheese on top of each slice of bread.
- ! Sprinkle some cayenne or paprika powder on the sandwich halves and bake in the oven for about 15 minutes.
- ! Have some leafy greens with a drizzle of olive oil.

What to Do - Oopsie Bread

- ! Begin by separating the egg whites (whites in one bowl and yolks in the other).
- ! Whisk the egg whites with the salt until peaks are formed.
- ! Combine the cream cheese and egg yolks—add the baking powder and psyllium seed husk (making it more Oopsie type bread).
- ! Blend/fold in the whites into the yolk mixture—keeping out the air in the whites of the eggs.
- ! Place six or eight 'oopsie' on the paper-lined sheet.
- ! Bake in the middle rack of the oven at 300F until browned, usually for 25 minutes.

Dinner: Stuffed Poblanos

Total Prep & Cooking Time: 35 minutes

Yields: 4 Servings

Nutrition stats (one serving)

- Protein: 14 grams
- Net Carbs: 4 grams
- Fats: 36 grams
- Calories: 450

What to Use

! Bacon fat (1 T)

! Pork (1 lb. ground)

! Onion (.5)

! Poblano peppers (4)

! Baby belle mushrooms (7)

! Cumin (1 tsp.)

! Vine tomato (1 tsp.)

! Chili powder (1 tsp.)

! Cilantro (.25 c chopped)

! Salt (as desired)

! Pepper (as desired)

What to Do

! Rinse and prep all the vegetables, you want to mince garlic, slice the mushrooms and onions, and dice the tomatoes. If your cilantro is not already chopped, do this as well.

! Set your oven to broil, while this is heating up, place the poblanos on a cookie sheet and put them in the oven when it is hot. Broil them for around 8 to 10 minutes, make sure to move them around every two minutes, you want consistent marks over the entire pepper. Then preheat your oven to 350F.

! Using a paper towel or gloves to cover your fingers, carefully pull the skin from the peppers. Also, set the skin aside.

! In a pan that is set on medium high-heat, begin to cook the pork, this is also where you add the bacon fat. Season with salt and pepper, but do not taste it until it has cooked all the way.

! When it is browned you may now add the chili powder and cumin.

! In the pan, slide all of the pork to one side

and add the garlic and onions to the other side, you want them to be softened.

! When those have softened add the mushrooms and mix all of it together, add more salt and pepper to suit your palate.

! When the mixture starts to dry out a little add the tomatoes and cilantro.

! Make a slice in the poblano pepper from the bottom to the stem and use a spoon or your fingers to remove the seeds. The seeds are spicy, so if you are sensitive to spicy foods, be sure to remove all of them.

! Carefully fill each pepper with the pork mixture and bake them for around 8 to 10 minutes.

! Remove them from the oven and they are now ready to serve!

Chapter 6:

Adding in Intermittent Fasting

Fasting can sound scary. You might have had to fast for blood work at the doctor and been absolutely famished by the time your blood was drawn. You might have read of long 40 day fasts in some religions. You might be wondering what in the world a chapter about fasting is doing in a book about building up your fat intake.

Adding intermittent fasting to your new lifestyle is the final step in turning your body into an absolute fat burning machine. When you fast, your body naturally burns more fat when it is not dealing with elevated glucose levels, which is something you are not going to have to worry much about while on the keto diet. As such, by putting these two together you maximize your fat burning effectiveness. This means, if you are really looking to lose as much weight as possible you are going to want to work intermittent fasting into your plan.

Conventional wisdom says that breakfast is the most important meal of the day because it gets your metabolism going. The principles behind intermittent fasting say that breakfast is the worst meal of the day because it activates hormones that lead to weight gain. When your body is digesting and absorbing the nutrients from food, it is in what is called a fed state. This fed state begins when you take your first bite and ends about three to five hours later, which is usually about the time when you will eat again. During a fed state, your insulin levels are high, so your body will not burn much fat if any at all.

No matter how much you watch what you eat, how few carbs you consume, or how much you exercise, you will not lose much weight if your body is stuck in a high-insulin cycle. This is because insulin is a hormone that is secreted to help regulate your blood sugar by causing it to be absorbed by your body's cells. What does the absorbed blood sugar turn into? Fat. If your blood has too much sugar in it, insulin will signal your liver to absorb it in the form of... fat. In other words, when your body is in a fed state, it is perpetually creating fat, no matter what you may be doing to try to burn it.

The way it works is that sometime between 2 and 8 hours after you eat your last meal, your body enters a state of fasting. While your body is in this state, your blood sugar (or glucose) level drops to a more tolerable threshold. This also reduces the amount of insulin floating through your bloodstream. When your glucose level drops and stabilizes a bit, a hormone called glucagon is released from your liver. Once the glucagon is released into the bloodstream, its job is to release the stored energy in your cells. This raises the glucose levels in your bloodstream, which are primarily used as fuel by the brain and red blood cells.

Once these storage tanks of glucose are emptied, your body goes in search of alternative fuel sources. Since there is not enough glucose for fuel, your body begins to break down its fat cells, supercharging your weight loss in the process.

There are very few negative side-effects with every intermittent fasting method. The greatest concern that participants typically encounter is a short- term feeling of hunger and lulls in energy levels. However, this concern is short- lived and is generally uncommon with fasting.

Many people are afraid that they will spend their entire morning feeling miserable because they have not eaten yet. But most participants don't experience any negative side-effects and actually even experience increased energy and overall better health. Fasting gives your cells time to repair themselves and grow so that your body can heal and improve your immune system.

Before you begin an intermittent fasting plan, you should check with your physician to be sure you are physically fit. These are some of the elements to consider:

- ! History of eating disorders

- ! Have diabetes

- ! If you are too thin/underweight

- ! Have low blood pressure

- ! Currently taking prescribed or non-prescribed medications

- ! Have issues with regulation of your blood sugar

- ! Female with amenorrhea history

- ! Female actively attempting to become pregnant

- ! Breastfeeding or pregnant

- ! History of eating disorders

Fasting benefits

Simplifies your schedule: Reducing stress, simplicity, and behavioral changes can all combine to change your life in an amazing way. Intermittent fasting gives you more simplicity, making life more open for what you truly enjoy.

When you wake in the morning, you won't have to worry about making breakfast, you can just drink some water and begin the day. Eating is nice, and cooking is fun for some people, so eating thrice daily isn't always a hassle, but intermittent fasting frees up a chunk of time that would've otherwise been dedicated to food in some way. Life gets simpler which means less stress.

Repair your digestive tract: There are many foods in today's world that contain refined carbohydrates, additives, preservatives, chemicals, and other ingredients that are not only difficult for your body to break down, but also cause more stress on your digestive system. Over time, your digestive tract does not function properly; making food more difficult to digest and resulting in conditions such as irritable bowel syndrome. Fasting will allow your digestive system to repair and rebalance so it can better fight off toxins.

Lowers risk of cancer: Whether or not intermittent fasting can help to reduce cancer risks is still being debated since there isn't enough research to prove it. But the reports at this time do seem promising. One study of 10 different cancer sufferers suggested that chemotherapy side effects could be diminished by pretreatment fasting. What was found here also appears to be supported by a study that instructed cancer patients to fast every other day and showed that this resulted in fewer deaths and better cure rates. Lastly, a comprehensive analysis of disease and fasting has shown that fasting may reduce cancer risks along with cardiovascular disease.

Give your liver a break: Your liver is another organ that regularly removes toxins from the body and process food products that contain tons of nutrients that take time and energy to break down. Your liver is the primary organ for cleansing the body. Every food molecule that you consume and is absorbed through the intestinal wall will first go through your liver to be prepped for utilization. Fasting allows your liver to rest and regenerate new cells that will improve its overall function.

Rest your stomach: Your stomach is put under constant stress when consuming three or more meals a day and is overloaded with processed foods and chemicals on a daily basis. There are millions of people around the world who rely on acid-suppressing medicines or cannot produce enough acid to help break down food. Simply allowing your stomach to rest by not eating for a little will allow it to heal, function properly, and reset your digestive system.

Increase your lifespan: Scientific studies have been proving for a long time that calorie restriction is effective for lengthening the lifespan. Logically, this does make perfect sense. When your body is starving, it figures out how to extend its own existence. But there's an issue here. Does anyone really want to go through starving themselves just to live longer? Life should be enjoyable, not completely miserable. Fortunately, intermittent fasting calls to action a lot of the same functions that extend life as restricting calories. To put it another way, you will get the advantage of living longer, without having to starve yourself. One particular study done in 1945 proved that mice that did intermittent fasting lived longer.

Intermittent Fasting's Effect on Type 2 Diabetes: Sadly, type 2 diabetes is not uncommon and has developed in a stronger way recently. The most common symptom of this disease is blood sugar imbalances in a way that relates to your body's insulin resistance. When insulin resistance is lessened, this helps lower blood sugar levels and protects you against this disease. Intermittent fasting has been proven to offer large benefits for the body's resistance to insulin and thus helps reduce blood sugar levels.

In some research done on intermittent fasting in humans, blood sugar levels during a fast went down as much as 6 percent, and insulin was lowered over 30 percent. A study done with diabetic rats proved that intermittent fasting could reduce kidney damage, which matters because this is a side effect of advanced diabetes. In other words, based on these studies, intermittent fasting could be highly significant for those at risk of type 2 diabetes.

But keep in mind that there may be some differences in terms of type 2 diabetes, fasting, and gender. A study showed that for females, blood sugar control actually worsened when intermittent fasting was done for over 20 days. In other words, intermittent fasting shows great promise in helping type 2 diabetes, but it seems more advantageous for men.

Limitations on fasting

Most people are able to safely fast, but as with

anything else, some exceptions exist. Most of the time, all you have to have in order to fast safely is decent and average health.

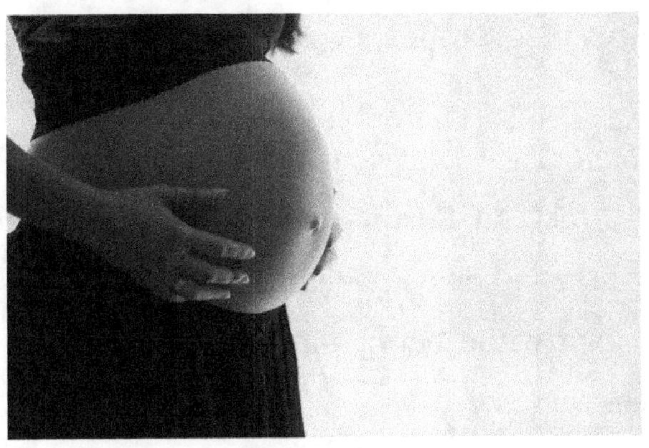

Nursing or pregnant women: The impacts of fasting on pregnancy are not yet known. In terms of nursing, it is believed that your milk has fewer nutrients during a fast than it has when you are following normal eating patterns. Therefore, it may be harmful to your baby.

Those with certain medical problems: As said before, you shouldn't do fasting if you have some diseases or weaknesses in the kidneys or liver. In addition, you should not fast if you're generally exhausted, anemic, malnourished, or frail. You should ask your doctor or be supervised by a professional during fasts if you have high blood pressure, a weak immune system, diabetes that requires medications, or a fainting problem.

Children: In America, it's not recommended for kids to fast. In Europe, however, it's considered okay if the kid is overweight and chose the fast on their own while being watched over by a health professional.

After a major sickness or surgery: You should take some time to fully recover before you try to do any fasting. Fasting should generally be done when you are feeling relatively strong and not wiped out by a recent surgery or illness.

Those with an eating disorder history: If you have had bulimia or anorexia in the past, it's generally advised that you do not fast.

With some conditions, you can still fast, but if the condition is very serious, you may need the support of a doctor to make sure it's safe for you. If you are taking some medications, the health requirements could vary for that medicine, so having a doctor monitor you during a fast is recommended. Anyone who is uncertain about the idea of fasting should ask a doctor before starting.

Important Note: Keep in mind, nothing is considered risky or dangerous in intermittent fasting, but it is always best to be sure you are healthy before you make any major changes in your diet needs. Remember the most common consequence using this procedure is hunger—not starvation. You might experience some mood swings and want to over-eat when you are on your days off, but the plans are healthy. You also, will not starve!

Chapter 7:

Know Your Types of Intermittent Fasting

16/8 Method: This method involves fasting for either 16 hours for men or 14 hours for women before allowing yourself to consume a reasonable amount of calories for the 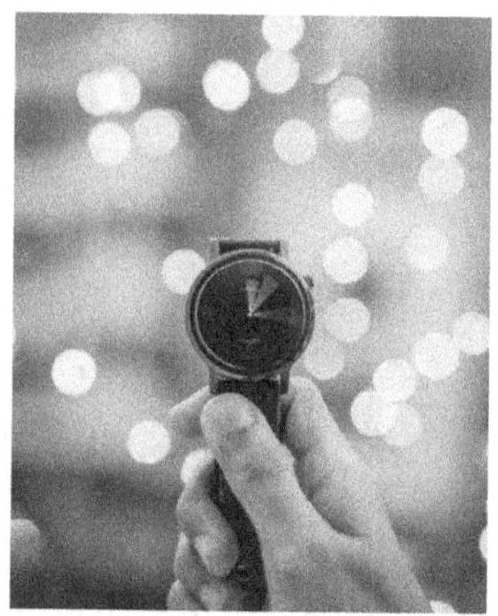 remaining 8 to 10 hours. During this period, you should only consume things that have zero calories including black coffee (a splash of cream is fine), water, diet soda, and sugar-free gum. The easiest way to attempt this schedule is to stop eating after dinner in the evening and wait 14 or 16 hours from there. This means skipping breakfast and picking things up in the early afternoon.

This type of intermittent fasting is one of the most flexible options available which means it can work well for just about everyone. Many people find that they can comfortably eat 2 filling meals in the 8 or 10 hours they have to consume calories or, even three regular meals in a shortened time frame. The important thing is to find a method that works with you and stick with it long term.

Most people who stick to the 16/8 split stop eating after a filling dinner and then eat a somewhat late lunch before starting the cycle all over again. This doesn't mean you have to stick to this split, however, and indeed, one of the best parts of any intermittent fasting lifestyle is the inherent flexibility. For example, if you exercise first thing in the morning then you may want to break your fast after you are finished to provide your body the fuel it needs to build strong muscles. It is recommended that you factor the period you are asleep into your timetable as doing so is more likely to lead to success.

Whatever time table you choose, it is important that it does what it can to promote your success, as opposed to being something you have to actively struggle against. The goal should be to follow the same eating schedule every day to maximize your results by getting your body into the habit of burning fat during a specific period each day. If you vary when you are fasting too regularly, it can throw your hormones out of whack, which in turn, can make it much more likely that your body will hold on to, as opposed to shedding, those extra pounds.

If you find that you are having trouble getting started at first, then this may be because you are trying to force an ineffective eating schedule upon yourself. When you decide what time period is going to frame your fast, it is important to choose the time period that makes it easiest for you to go without for as long as possible, rather than one you have to struggle against for sixteen straight hours. Lock it in once you find it, however, as this is the only way you will be able to accurately determine how much weight this type of fasting allows you to burn.

If you find yourself in a situation where you will not be able to realistically break your fast as you normally would, it is important to prepare for this fact as best you can and do whatever is in your power to keep your new normal going as much as possible. With that being said, it isn't the end of the world if you happen to eat a single meal outside of your standard eight or ten hours. If this occurs simply start your fast as normal at the end of the day and keep yourself on track as much as possible.

If you find yourself really struggling with the final few hours of your fast, then this is likely because you are not consuming an adequate amount of protein in the time you have allotted yourself to break your fast. During your eight or ten hours you are going to want to consume 55 grams of protein per day for women and 60 grams each day for min. Not only will this help you stick to your fasts more readily, but it will help you build plenty of healthy muscle as well.

Warrior Method: If you are looking for an intermittent fasting variant that is between the 16:8 method and the eat, stop, eat method then the warrior method has you covered. For this type of intermittent fasting, you spend 20 hours of the day fasting and then consume your daily caloric requirements in the remaining 4 hours. The first meal you consume should include about 65 percent of your daily caloric intake and the second should take up the remaining 35 percent.

The basis for this type of intermittent fasting comes from the idea that ancient humans hunted at night which meant they spent a majority of their time in a fasting state. This fact leads proponents of the warrior method to posit that the human body is more poised to absorb nutrients properly by simply eating in a condensed window at the end of the day. The idea here is that by eating during this window you will end up feeling fuller while still consuming a smaller number of calories overall.

While this might sound like a bit of a stretch, the science behind it is surprisingly sound. You see, every night when the sun goes down, this transition causes the human body's fight or flight response to activate because the lack of readily available light means it is more difficult to identify threats. This change is felt throughout the body and one of the side effects is that you will naturally burn more fat from the foods you eat during this time.

For those who feel as though they won't be able to go 20 hours between meals, the warrior diet actually allows for 1 serving of dark, leafy green vegetables as well as 30 grams of protein. The best way to take advantage of this fact is to consume the vegetables prior to exercising and the protein afterwards to give you extra energy and help you build muscles respectively. When you do end up breaking your fast in full you will want to start with a meal that is high in healthy fats and nutrient rich.

When you break your fast at night, you must eat particular food groups in a particular order. First, you eat broth, then vegetables, protein/meat, and then fat. Eating at night maximizes the parasympathetic nervous system, which helps the body to recuperate, become calm, relax, digest while the body uses the nutrients for growth and for repair. It may also help the body to produce fat-burning hormones that work on your fat the next day.

Another aspect of this diet is to do strength training during the days. Do squats, pull-ups, high jumps, press-ups, frog jumps, and sprints. Select three of these activities, doing two sets of five minutes each during a thirty-minute period of time that you set aside every day. Drink a protein shake before you exercise.

A person who can regularly follow this diet will

turn his or her body into a fat-burning and muscle-forming machine! One also gets to eat something during the fasting time, which helps the person endure the fasting hours. People experience increased energy and greater loss of fat when they adopt this eating style.

However, the strict schedule and eating guidelines are hard for some people to follow, especially if they have to attend a lot of social gatherings. Additionally, some people prefer to not eat large meals late at night.

5:2 Fasting: Another common intermittent fasting protocol is the 5:2 diet. This particular protocol involves normal eating for five days per week then restricting calorie intake for two days of the week. This protocol was made popular by a British doctor and journalist, Michael Mosley.

This protocol is more of an eating pattern than an actual diet. It requires women to restrict their calorie intake to 500 on fasting days. First, identify two non-consecutive days of the week and mark them as fast days. For instance, Monday and Thursday are preferred by most people.

On regular days, you should eat normally and without bingeing. You should also avoid junk foods as these will erode the great benefits of the fast. Plenty of women find this protocol much easier to follow than traditional diets.

Studies surrounding this type of intermittent fasting show that it is likely to lead to an increased insulin resistance for those with diabetes, reduce the risk of heart arrhythmia, reduction of hot flashes and relief from both seasonal allergies and asthma. Additionally, a 12-week study of those using the 4:3 method revealed that the average practitioner saw a reduce in fat mass by 3.5 kg with no negative impact to muscle mass and an overall body weight reduction of 5 kg which came along with a 20 percent reduction in triglycerides and overall lower levels of blood pressure.

Perhaps most impressive, those who follow this type of intermittent fasting tend to see up to 40 percent lower leptin levels than normal. Additionally, they saw reduced levels of CRP which is a maker that indicates overall levels of inflammation in the body.

As with all types of intermittent fasting, it is extremely important to avoid overindulging on the days that you are eating freely as it is extremely easy to eat 500 to 600 calories without even realizing it. If you keep it up, however, you will eventually be able to train your body to expect a diet that is more well-structured to ensure that you don't feel as hungry on your fast days. Think carefully about the foods you eat on these days as 500 calories can either be a handful of Oreos or a lightly seasoned fish filet and one will help you make it through far more easily than the other.

The 4:3 plan also recommends that you skip breakfast and measure your weight daily. For those whose weight tends to fluctuate more than average this is not recommended, however, as it can be disheartening without actually proving much one way or the other.

Alternate-Day Fasting: The alternate-day fasting is another type of intermittent fasting. On this diet, you fast every other day, and then you eat whatever you want on non-fasting days. A modified version of this protocol involves eating about 500 calories on fasting days.

Alternate-day fasting is considered a very effective method of losing weight and also helps with numerous other health benefits as well. Your eating is restricted only half the time, yet the benefits are immense. During fasting days, you are allowed to drink as many beverages as you wish as long as they are calorie-free. For instance, you can have water, unsweetened tea, green tea, and coffee.

On the modified alternative-day fast, you are

allowed to consume 20 – 25 percent of your energy requirements which is about 500 calories. Studies also indicate that women prefer this protocol compared to old-fashioned diets because the fast is broken each day and they get to choose foods that they like.

When you first start this form of intermittent fasting the easiest way to make it through the low calorie days is by trying any one of a variety of protein shakes. It is important to work back to real natural foods on these days as they will always be healthier than the shakes. This form of intermittent fasting is all about losing weight and those who try it tend to average between two and three pounds lost per week. If you attempt the Alternate Day Diet, it is extremely important to eat regularly on your full-calorie days as binge will not only negate any progress you will have made but it can also cause serious damage to your body if kept up over time.

The biggest downside to this type of intermittent

fasting is that you don't get the benefits of entering a true fasted state. However, limiting your calories is still going to help you moderate your weight more easily while also helping you get in the habit of restricting your diet, putting you in a spot where you can more easily control your eating habits with a more traditional form of fasting in the future. If you are unsure of just how many calories you are consuming in a given day, it is important to always err on the side of consuming less than consuming more as hitting this 20 percent is key to seeing weight loss results. With that being said, it is important to hone in on just how many calories you need as perpetually consuming too few calories can lead to malnutrition which can, in turn, lead to long lasting bodily damage.

A large number of people find this a very easy way to practice a variation of intermittent fasting in the long-term. So much so that it has nearly twice as many long-term adherents than any other type of intermittent fasting. What's more, you will likely see as much as 3 pounds of weight loss per week as your body transitions to this new way of eating.

Eat-Stop-Eat: With this type of intermittent fasting you will want to fast for 24 hours either once or twice a week. Once or twice each week, you will fast for twenty-four hours. As an illustration, you would eat dinner one morning and not eat again until the following morning. Most professionals say if you make it to twenty hours; it is okay. To further condition your body, for two days eat about 2,500 calories if you are a man and 2,000 if you are a woman. After several regular eating days, attempt another fasting, and repeat the agenda.

For the days on an active fast, try not consume many calories. You can drink sparkling or plain water, diet soda, coffee, or tea. When the fast is complete, eat what you like using restraint. Enjoy plenty of veggies, fruits, and take advantage of the spices for variety.

Protein should be apparent using twenty to thirty grams of high-quality protein. Consume a total of one-hundred grams every four to five hours. You can use protein powders if needed. If you are gaining extra pounds during in between your fasting schedule, consider cutting back by approximately 10% on the amount of food you consume on non-fasting days.

Some individuals cannot 'hack' the plan and state it makes them less adaptable to enjoying time with friends at social gatherings. Many have issues of crankiness and headaches which can lead to the plan's failure.

With that said, the plan's benefits are overwhelming because you can judge your progress, and you choose to eat. It takes learning some self-control, but you can get it. Never fast for two consecutive days. Also, you should not take the challenge more than two fasting days in one week.

With a strict plan such as this one, you must remain hydrated. You can drink plenty of clear liquids but where are the nutrients. On your fasting days, stick to apple juice water, broth, cranberry juice, ice pops, plain gelatin, black coffee or tea. This is okay since you will be fasting for twenty to twenty-four hours.

Ultimate Fat Loss and Muscle Gain: The most popular program based on this method is Leangains, which was created to help dedicated athletes and weight lifters lose body fat and build muscle. During this method, women fast for fourteen hours each day, and men fast for sixteen hours. While fasting, you are not allowed to consume any calories. However, you are allowed to drink black coffee, sugar- free gum, water, black tea, and calorie- free sweeteners. And, truth be told, adding a splash of creamer into your morning cup of coffee isn't going to hurt. The remaining eight to ten hours of your day represent your feasting period. Most participants of this method will find that fasting throughout the night and well into the morning is the easiest way to follow this intermittent fast. For this practice, the first meal is typically consumed about six hours after waking up. This fasting-feasting cycle is easy to adapt into any lifestyle, however, consistency with the feasting window is important. This is important because your hormones can be affected if you do not adhere to a strict program.

When and what you eat within the feasting period is entirely dependent on when you exercise. During the days you exercise, complex carbohydrates are more important than consuming fat; as you need the quick energy to prepare and recover from your work out. On your rest days, you should consume a lower number of carbs and a high amount of fat. Throughout the week, your protein intake should be relatively high, depending on your goals, gender, body fat percentage, etc. Regardless of your chosen workout regiment, your diet should be mostly made up of whole, unprocessed, foods that will adequately nourish your body.

Chapter 8:

Start Off Fasting on the Right Foot

Ages ago, people looked at fasting as a form of supreme sacrificing, as a punishment even. Fasting was a way to rid their bodies of carnal needs and spiritual temptations. In fact, fasting was often coupled with flogging as a form of self-punishment. It's no wonder many people perceive fasting as a negative, available to those who prefer self-deprivation to self-acceptance and forgiveness. They've never thought of fasting as a way to gain greater insight and knowledge, to bring about physical and emotional healing, or as a way to increase strength and energy.

So, before you make a commitment to fast, pause for a few moments to consider how you feel about fasting. Does the thought of fasting excite you? Do you anticipate positive changes to happen after having successfully fasted? If you cannot see fasting in a positive light, then perhaps it is not for you. Fasting is to some like running a marathon is to others. Some people have not experienced the altered state one moves into when they are a few miles into a long marathon. They have never felt first-hand the new rhythm and satisfaction you get when you let go of the thoughts of how much your muscles are straining and begin to think about ways to live a better life helping others.

Fasting offers that same escape. If you can make yourself stop fantasizing about food and think of a deeper purpose and meaning to your life, the distractions begin to fade away, and your commitment to the fast takes center stage. You get into the zone, and then, without a doubt, you just know you will finish your fast and succeed in achieving your purpose—and then some. It's amazing how your senses become much more intense when you are fasting. If you can't focus on your purpose, concentrate on how you are experiencing the world differently through your heightened sensitivity.

Here are some steps to help you get started including intermittent fasting with your keto diet:

Don't go all the way up front: Don't try to intermittent fast in the first weeks of a ketogenic diet or if you follow the Standard American Diet. This is extremely important. Your body needs to get adapted to keto before you try intermittent fasting. Your body must get used to eating low-carbs so your body can utilize ketones for energy instead of using glucose. If you try intermittent fasting at the same time you begin the keto diet, you will not succeed. You will be too glucose-dependent and too hungry to stick with it. There is some misinformation around about intermittent fasting. Intermittent fasting needs to be natural and not a struggle, and you should never feel hungry. It will be a gradual process and take time before it is used effectively.

Listen to your body: You must listen to your body. Intermittent fasting works best if it is done naturally. If you realize it's lunchtime, but you don't feel hungry, just skip it and eat at dinner time. If it is too late to eat? Skip dinner and eat breakfast. Most people find it easier to skip breakfast anyway. Try to eat about 1 pm and eat again about four hours before you go to bed, so your body has time to digest your foods.

Start slow: Don't force yourself to do intermittent fasting. You should never deprive or restrict yourself. When your body has become fat-adapted, you won't feel as hungry. Begin by staying away from snacks between meals. Next, try skipping regular meals. Do this only if you don't feel hungry.

Stay busy: You might find it easier to skip meals if you are busy and don't spend time in the kitchen. You might be tempted to have a snack if you are around food, even if you don't feel hungry. It is easy to go without food when you are out shopping. Remember to drink plenty of liquid. Water, tea, or coffee is all you need.

Try it for at least a month: You need at least three to four weeks to determine if the intermittent fast is right for you. If you don't do it for this long, then you are not giving the body the time it needs to adapt, and you are not giving it a fair shot. Try it out for at least this amount of time to see if it's the right choice for you

Restrain yourself: When you do eat during your fast, do not entirely throw nutrition out the window. Consider food quality and eat "normally." While there are no strict die-hard dietary rules to some fasting plans, and that's not so much the point, but the best results will usually be received if you are eating normally when you do eat, rather than trying to make up for lost calories during the fast. You will want to eat until you are full, not until you feel nauseous and over-fed, and focus on consuming carbs rather than unhealthy fats.

While normal eating is mostly encouraged, other fasters like to include one "cheat day" during their feeding times, where they indulge in absolutely anything they want, no matter what that is. Cheat days like these work because they encourage the mind as a sort of reward system for tirelessly eating healthy the rest of the week, but the effect is not solely on your psyche. Fat cells release a hormone called leptin to helps maintain energy in the body. This is what you are feeling signal you to stop eating when you feel full and satisfied with your meal, once your body acknowledges that it has sufficient energy stored and is ready to go.

When leptin levels dip, you might feel ravenous, and this is often times the culprit behind binge eating or overeating on well-meaning diets. The longer calorie intake is restricted, and fatty foods are avoided, the lower these levels dip and a "diet breaker" is generally inevitable at some point in the near future because of these leptin hormones making you feel terribly hungry. Also, restricting calories can lower the thyroid hormones that help maintain your metabolic rate and contribute to bone health. This decrease in metabolism is rather counter-productive while dieting, and some fasters believe a cheat day helps to balance this out and keep everything functioning well.

Play around with fasting methods: What works for one person may not work for you. If you find that certain fasting times are better or that a particular version of intermittent fasting is more effective, then choose those. It's all experimenting to see what feels right for you. Every diet is going to have periods of weight loss plateau, that is simply a part of weight loss that cannot be mitigated. As long as you stay consistent weight loss will eventually resume. The worst thing you can do is to try and change things up to get weight loss back on track as that will only make it more difficult for your body to start shedding weight once more. Instead, if you stay the course and keep up the good work you will start seeing results again before you know it.

Avoid the bad stuff: You need to make sure that you are not using it as an excuse to eat junk food

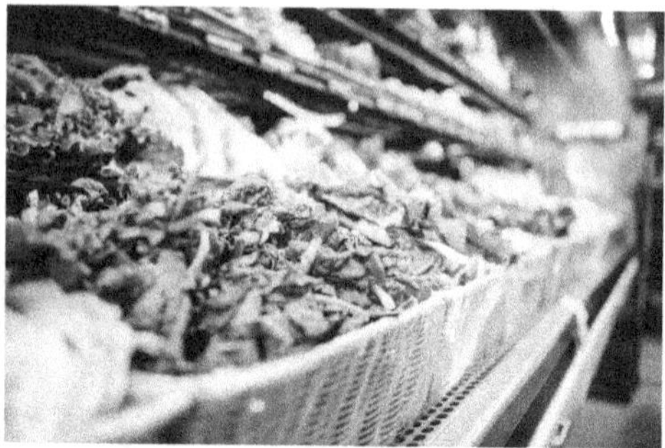

all the time. Make sure to stick with a well-balanced diet so that you provide your body with enough nutrition, even if you choose to go on a fast. It is important to keep in mind that a big part of intermittent fasting is building up a calorie defect by the end of the week to support additional weight loss. As such, if you fill your body full of high-calorie junk food when you do enter an eating window, what you are really doing is undoing all of your hard work. Making healthy choices at all times will improve the overall effectiveness of your weight loss efforts, guaranteed.

Understand delayed gratification: Delayed gratification works well at the onset of your new lifestyle. Think of it as the situation where a child requests its mother to go outside and play. Instead of saying a direct yes, the mother puts it off until a little later. This delay eases the hunger and pain of desire. Similarly, always try and approach intermittent fasting this way. When you think about the sumptuous meal awaiting you, try and delay it for an hour or two until you learn to ignore it completely until the right time.

Sometimes, your workmates or the people you live with will offer you drinks or snacks. Delicious chocolate, ice-cream, milkshakes, and so on are likely to tempt you. While these are pretty tempting, consider applying the principle of delayed gratification to stave off your desire to eat until later. If you can successfully repel such temptations, write it down in a diary as a reminder of the impressive progress you are making.

Stick to the plan: When you put so much time and effort into making a plan for your fasting it is that much easier to stick to it when the time comes. After all, if you don't stick to your plan, that's a lot of wasted time and effort. However, plans can change, and you must be ready and willing to roll with the punches.

For example, you might get to the conference center on a business trip and discover that the itinerary has completely changed from what you were told in advance. They may now be offering food during your fasting periods. Use your willpower to avoid breaking your fast too early. Find other activities to do away from the offered food if possible, or simply politely turn it down.

You might get to a restaurant and find that the menu you found online isn't accurate, and you aren't able to stick to your calorie restrictions. When this happens, you might not have the time to find another restaurant with a healthier menu. Instead, go ahead and get the healthiest item possible that you will enjoy. If you go significantly over your planned calorie intake, simply start your fast immediately after the meal instead of a couple of hours later. For instance, if you are eating from 12:00 p.m. to 8:00 p.m. and you're having the dinner at 6:00 p.m., start your fast at 7:00 p.m. instead of 8:00 p.m. You might add an hour or two to the other end of your fast as well.

Be prepared for things to change, but to stick to your overall plan regardless of the changes in your schedule and menu. This will help you be more successful with your intermittent fasting so that you can continue to work on your weight loss goals while traveling.

Other things you can do: You can take a photo just before you begin this lifestyle change so that in the weeks and months to come, you will note the amazing changes that will take place. Such photos and the notable changes will motivate you especially as you embark on this crucial lifestyle change.

As you fast and also workout, your body will release more HGH or human growth hormone.

This hormone will enable your body to develop strong, lean muscles that are toned and well developed. A progress photo will serve as an excellent motivation tool and will keep you focused on your intermittent fasting journey.

The bottom line: At the end of the day it is important to appreciate and understand just what it is you are undertaking and what you are expecting out of your body. Much like the keto diet, adding intermittent fasting to your dietary habits is a lifestyle change more than it is a temporary diet. As a lifestyle, it has the potential to make you into a better person mentally, physically and psychologically. While the going will be tough at first, once you make it through the initial month you will find that the benefits have been so substantial that you have no desire to turn back.

Chapter 9:

Intermittent Fasting and Exercise

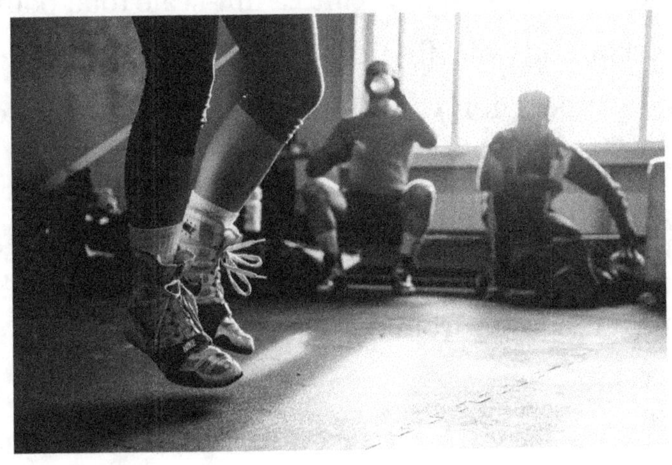

It doesn't matter if you are training for endurance or training to improve your strength, your body primarily uses the glycogen found in stored carbohydrates to fuel your exercise. However, when your glycogen reserves are running low, such as when you are in the latter half of a period of fasting, then your body is going to need to look to other energy sources like fat to power your exercise routine. This means that you are likely to burn up to 20 percent more fat if you exercise during a fast as opposed to just after you have broken one.

You don't have to jump into a full-scale total body workout on your first day, but simple things can do wonders for your level of fitness as you go along.

Try these steps to get you started and then build up your activity from there.

- Take the stairs rather than an elevator whenever you can. If you work in a high-rise building, it may not be feasible to climb 20 flights of stairs every time you go to work but maybe you can start by taking 1 flight and then gradually build up to taking more flights as you build up your strength and endurance. If you have stairs at home, consider going up and down them several times each time you have to use them. You'll burn off extra calories and you'll feel better at the same time.

- Start taking walks on your breaks and throughout the day. This is very important if you have a desk job. It will not only build up your endurance levels it will help to improve your posture and reduce stress, too. Get up every few hours and take a short walk around the building or around the block to help you burn off quite a few dormant calories.

- Consider getting a buddy to exercise with you. This is a great motivator and will be very helpful in keeping you on track. If you schedule a workout at the gym with your buddy you're less likely to find other things to do if you have a commitment. But you don't have to restrict your exercise to a gym. You can get some movement in when you go shopping, pick up your kids from school, or visit friends. Whatever you plan to do, leave with the mindset that you want to get your body moving, and something will come up.

Taking it up a notch

The following exercise routines can be mixed and matched depending on which you like the most. Make a concentrated effort to hit the major muscles groups in each workout including arms, abs, legs, chest, and back. Taking the time to focus on each area, every time you exercise will ensure you eventually see full body results. When you start, make a point of exercising at least three times per week.

Remember, it is unreasonable to expect major results after just a month (or less) of exercising regularly. Consider how long it took for you to become the way you are now and cut your body some slack, you will see results sooner than you may think. While performing each of the following routines it is important to spend as little time resting in between individual exercises as possible to maximize results. This month will set the tone for all of the months to come, make it count.

No equipment full body routine: Run down the list 4 times in a row while allowing yourself up to 3 minutes to rest between attempts. Feel free to take up to 45 seconds to rest between each exercise but do not take more time than you need to move on as the goal is to finish the list as quickly as possible.

- Start by holding plank as long as possible
- Perform 8 squats
- Perform 8 lunges
- Perform 8 pushups
- Perform 8 leg raises
- Perform as many mountain climbers as possible
- Perform 8 pike pushups

Full body routine: Run down the list 3 times in a row while allowing yourself up to 4 minutes to rest between attempts. Feel free to take up to 1 minute to rest between each exercise but do not take more time than you need to move on as the goal is to finish the list as quickly as possible.

- Start by performing 3 chinups
- Perform a wall sit for 30 seconds
- Perform 12 dips using a chair
- Perform 8 squats
- Perform 8 pushups
- Perform 2 pullups
- Perform 3 leg raises
- Perform 7 decline pushups

Exercise options

Don't overdo it: Exercise by itself does not lead to an increase in strength or dexterity, exercising by itself only breaks your muscles down. You must include a recovery period in your exercise regime in order to see the most results. As such, even when you have master the advanced exercises listed in chapter five, you should plan to take at least one day off a week from bodyweight exercises to give your body the time it needs to make the most of the gift you are giving it every time you exercise.

Over training alone will not destroy your muscles, even after extreme strain they will repair themselves completely given about a week's time. However, over training can lead to serious or even permanent damage to the tendons and ligaments. Tendons are responsible for attaching bone to muscle while ligaments connect bones to other bones.

Innately ligaments and tendons are extremely strong but at the same time, they can take an extremely long time to heal properly. If you do not take the time to rest and recover between extensive periods of exercise you can develop tendonitis and your tendons will always be playing catchup. Continuing to work through the pain of tendonitis you can develop permanent disabilities in the form of tendonitis.

Many bodyweight exercises put undue stress on the shoulders which is why you will want to always take note of how your shoulders are feeling and ensure you do not push them too far. Young people may feel as though they can keep going indefinitely but it is important to remember that the goal when exercising regularly is to continue to do so for many years to come.

Keep it low-intensity: If you hope to exercise throughout the fasting process then it is important that you keep things low-intensity while you are fasting. This means you are going to want to ensure you can carry on a normal conversation while in the midst of doing whatever it is you are doing. This is something mild like 10 minutes on a stationary bike or a light jog, anything that doesn't push you past your limits.

While exercising it will be extremely important to take the time to listen to the signals your body is providing you with and to take a break if things start to take a turn. Keep in mind that you will be running on far less fuel than normal which means it is possible you may become dizzy or get light-headed more quickly than you would in most other instances. If you make the mistake of ignoring what your body is trying to tell you then it is only going to end up making the rest of your time exercising all the more unmanageable.

Timing is everything: When it comes to getting the most out of each exercise session, specifically if you are looking to push yourself to your limits, then the best time to do so is going to be about 60 minutes after you have broken your last fast. This will give your body the time it needs to start processing food for energy so that you have what you need in order to push yourself to the limit. It doesn't matter if you are fasting every day or only a few times a week, taking this into account will allow you to ensure your muscles will have all the fuel they need to grow and repair themselves after each session.

Make a choice: While eating before exercising is the right choice if you are looking to steadily build muscle if you are looking to lose as much weight as you possibly can you will want to exercise on an empty stomach instead. You won't want to go at it as vigorously, however, and instead stick to something light like a low-intensity jog or a beginner's spin class. You will still want to schedule this close to the time when you will be breaking your fast, however, as your body will be very demanding afterwards and expect the fuel it needs to keep things running at maximum efficiency.

It will also require planning ahead during your previous eating period as you will want to load up on extra fat to ensure your body has the fuel it needs to make it through all that cardio. As long as you can ensure your exercise needs meet your current level of nutrition then you should be on the right track.

Approach things properly: As a general rule, there is not upper limit when it comes to the amount of exercise you can undertake while fasting, as long as you keep regularly listening to your body. This should prevent you from overdoing it and pushing yourself harder than you should. Luckily, some studies show that strength levels continue to increase up to 16 hours after entering a fasted state. Nevertheless, you will want to take things slow to start as you can always increase the intensity later but you risk hurting yourself if you do too much too soon.

If you are looking to push yourself to the limit then it is important to add extra protein to your diet to ensure your muscles can continue to grow. Likewise, if you find yourself feeling nauseous or weak then this is a surefire indicator that you aren't getting enough fat in your diet and your cells are looking for energy, something that can make it particularly difficult to make it through to your next meal. Finding the right mixture of exercise that strengthens the muscles without pushing them to the limit and burning the maximum amount of fat possible should be your ultimate goal. Trial and error is your friend here, don't be afraid to experiment.

If you are looking to take things to the extreme then you are definitely going to want to work out during your feeding period as you will be able to have a snack beforehand to fill up on fat and then a meal afterwards to reward your muscles with protein. If you prefer to workout in the mornings and still wish to fast as normal then you could move your eating window to start at 8 am.

Cardio: Studies show that if you are looking for an easy way to kickstart your weight loss during a plateau, an excellent way to do so is by prioritizing cardio on the days you are fasting and weight training on the days you are not. It is also known to decrease bad cholesterol and promote good cholesterol. Recommended cardio exercises with intermittent fasting for weight loss include;

! Cycling

! Running

! Jumping rope

! High intensity interval training is another great choice as it involves repeating a number of exercises in short bursts. If you are looking to maximize your workouts in a minimum amount of time, then this is a great place to start.

Weight training: Weight training can be successfully maintained while fasting regularly as long as you take the time to ensure your macros are on point to keep your body happy. Nevertheless, you are still going to want to take things more slowly as a rule as your body is already going to be running on fumes. Early on you will likely want to stick to cardio across all days until your body adapts to the intermittent fasting lifestyle.

As you won't have the energy for the average

varied exercise routine, you will want to keep your training sessions more intense and focused in order to ensure you see results. One ideal training strategy is known as the reverse pyramid which requires that you start with the most difficult set first to give your body the greatest amount of available energy to see it through to completion. Each set will then see that you become fatigued at an earlier point. This means you will be able to give it your all with every round as you will know there is no need to replicate it again which makes progress easier.

Regardless of how you plan on exercising it is vital that you start with a plan in mind and also track your progress. Doing so will make it easier to stay on track, especially on days where you are low on energy and you start thinking that skipping one day won't be the worst thing in the world. You will also be able to look back at what you have accomplished so far and see the results of all of your hard work.

Chapter 10:

Intermittent Fasting Tips for Success

Keep a food ledger and keep it balanced: Your daily calorie doesn't need to sit at a fixed amount, in fact, maintaining a healthy diet long term becomes significantly easier if you instead come to terms with the fact that you can't always plan every meal and snack and instead record what you do end up eating in a food ledger. A leger is different than a journal in that the goal of your food ledger should always be to balance it out to zero. If you overindulge for a day or two, balance your ledger by cutting back for a few days or exercising more. Carbs you eat should always be balanced out with either those you don't or additional exercise, no exceptions. Stick to a ledger and you can stick to a long-term healthy diet.

Grocery

shopping: Once you have a food plan in mind, grocery shopping should be a pretty straightforward experience. The biggest hurdle you will have to face, however, is going to be preparing for the unexpected. For example, you should be aware of a few different ingredient options for parts of dishes that you aren't sure your grocery store will stock. This will allow you to plan ahead effectively and make it easier to avoid making poor choices.

Mix things up: If you typically have a difficult time maintaining your weight loss goals, despite your best efforts, you may instead find it effective to mix up your daily routine to give new habits the time they need to take root. With these changes in place, you will find it is much easier to avoid whatever it is that you are trying to avoid, rather than staring at the hole it left in your schedule day in and day out. When it comes to creating a new, more disciplined, lifestyle, it is important to not bite off more than you can chew all at once. Instead, you are going to want to focus on adding discipline to one aspect of your life before moving on to the next.

Drink more water: Since you are adding new habits to your repertoire anyway, it is a good idea to add drinking more water to the list. Specifically, you should aim for about 64 ounces of water per day, to ensure your body has all the water it needs to operate at maximum efficiency. If you live in a warm, dry climate, or exercise regularly you are going to want to aim even higher and try and consume a gallon of water per day. If you don't drink that much water naturally or don't believe you need to drink the recommended amount, give it a try for a few weeks and you will be surprised by the results.

Specifically, you will be surprised at how frequently your body was sending you signals saying it was hungry when in reality it was just looking for something to drink. Drinking the right amount of water per day will also provide your metabolism with the boost that it needs to function in peak form and ensure you lose as much weight each week as possible. This is especially important as both intermittent fasting and remaining in ketosis are known to leave you more dehydrated than normal.

Drink the right caffeinated beverages: When consumed without any additives, both coffee and tea can help you jump-start your metabolism. The one thing you should never drink, however, is soda, even if it doesn't have any calories. The wide variety of artificial ingredients in diet sodas can have a wide variety of unpredictable effects on the body, including causing you to hold onto fat that you otherwise would have already ditched. Rather than stick with artificial stuff, you should focus on herbal teas such as Skinny Teatox which can really help you knock off the extra pounds. This is the case because the herbs in these teas are known to improve the rate at which your body metabolizes food while also decreasing the response that fat cells have to sugar. Finally, they are also known to improve the way that fat cells react to insulin which, in turn, helps to aid in digestion and increase the overall functionality of the metabolism.

When it comes to coffee, you should drink it black as the antioxidant catechins it contains have been proven to add a boost to the metabolic system. What's more, if you drink a double shot of espresso before you exercise you are likely to burn as many as 20 percent more calories than you would otherwise. You will see some benefit if you drink your cup of joe directly after exercising as well, though the effects will be lessened.

Build a routine: Regardless of your ultimate goals with intermittent fasting and the keto diet, if you aren't already maintaining a schedule where you can eat regularly, then it is important to make doing so a priority. Not only will eating at regular periods help you to feel better, but it will also ensure that your brain has the fuel required to make good decisions. Specifically, studies show that those with low blood sugar are three times more likely to make poor decisions based on a lack of resolve than those whose blood sugar was on point. Don't let something as simple as a lack of food trigger a relapse into behavior you are trying to avoid. Rather, make it a point of keeping healthy snacks on hand to ensure that you are always able to keep a clear head no matter what.

Begin each new day with a positive affirmation: An affirmation is a positive sentence which you take the time to write time and again throughout the day. A mantra basically the same thing but it is repeated throughout the day mentally instead. Affirmations and mantras are a great way to wean out background noise thoughts and effectively help retrain your brain and create new neural pathways. Some common affirmations or mantras include.

! My health is improving and so is my life.
! Today, I focus on the good things that are unfolding in my life.

! Trusting my body is becoming easier and easier.

! It's safe for me to be myself.

! Healing is happening in my body and in my mind.

! I am surrounded and protected in healing white light.

! Everything I eat heals me and nourishes me.

! Making small changes is becoming easier for me.

! Healing happens with each baby step I take.

! I am choosing progress over perfection.

! I am guided by my intuition. I know what to eat and how to live my life.

Plan ahead: Don't give an attack of craving sneak a chance up on you and make you break your fast early. Suspect getting ravenous and look forward to your day to check whether there are any circumstances or occasions where you'll wind up in a position to cheat. Prepare dinners and snacks that will hold you over until the point that your next meal time.

Stay true to yourself: While the wide variety inherent in intermittent fasting means that a wide variety of individuals are able to take advantage of its many benefits, this doesn't mean that it is the right choice for you right now. While you should still be able to make it through several fasts without incident after you have done so you will want to consider how you felt afterwards and how difficult it was for you to tow the line. You will also need to take into account what your natural habits are like when it comes to eating as well as your overall relationship with food once and for all. It will also be important to keep in mind that intermittent fasting is all about success in the long-term which means it is not the short-term solution you may be looking for.

It is its long-term nature that requires you to ask yourself if it is something you are going to be able to commit to in the long-term, if not with the first type of fasting you try then potentially with the second or even third. If you still have a long way to go when it comes to meeting your weight-loss goals then you may want to focus on maintaining the keto lifestyle fist, and then add in intermittent fasting when you are more able to deal with the additional requirements effectively. Starting off with something that has a steep learning curve like intermittent fasting can lead to mental blocks that make it more difficult to succeed in the future.

Don't expect results overnight: As you are going to be layering a secondary weight loss method on top of the keto diet, it can be easy to make the mistake of letting your expectations run away from you. It is important to avoid this temptation, however, as it is unreasonable to expect that something that took years to create (your body) can be instantly remade overnight.

For starters, it is unlikely that you are going to

lose much weight during the first week you start fasting, as your body will be busy trying to figure out what is going on. After that point, you will likely end up losing more weight than you were before for a time, but if you start to get close to your end goal then you will likely default to the standard one pound of fat lost per week which is the healthy average for prolonged weight loss.

Conclusion

Thanks for making it through to the end of *Intermittent Fasting and Ketogenic Diet: How you can adapt ketogenic diet and fasting to maximize fat loss and live healthy*, let's hope it was informative and able to provide you with all of the tools you need to achieve your weight loss goals, whatever it is that they may be. Just because you've finished this book doesn't mean there is nothing left to learn on the topic, and expanding your horizons is the only way to find the mastery you seek.

Now that you have finished this book, it is only natural to be extremely anxious to get started not only with the keto diet but with intermittent fasting as well. Nevertheless, it is important to follow the steps outlined in the following chapters and start with the keto diet before adding in intermittent fasting after your body has had the time it needs to adjust to the change, which should be a minimum of one month.

While you may be anxious to get started losing as much weight as possible, forcing your body to adapt to both lifestyle changes at once is likely to cause it to feel as though you are in a situation where it needs to hold on to every single calorie possible, curtailing weight loss in the process. Instead, it is important to give your body the time it needs to adjust and realize that following the ketogenic diet while fasting intermittently is more akin to a marathon than a sprint which means that slow and steady wins the race.

Finally, if you found this book useful in anyway, a review on Amazon is always appreciated!

www.ingramcontent.com/pod-product-compliance
Lightning Source LLC
Chambersburg PA
CBHW060046260726
48658CB00004B/1207